800 Days in Doha

800 Days in Doha

Penelope Gordon

CHAPLIN BOOKS

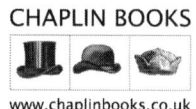

www.chaplinbooks.co.uk

Printed in the UK by Imprint Digital

Chaplin Books
5 Carlton Way
Gosport PO12 1LN
Tel: 023 9252 9020
www.chaplinbooks.co.uk

For Lionel. Thank you for sharing the adventures.

"I could tell you my adventures – beginning from this morning," said Alice a little timidly; "but it's no use going back to yesterday, because I was a different person then."
"Explain all that," said the Mock Turtle.
"No, no! The adventures first," said the Gryphon in an impatient tone; "explanations take such a dreadful time."

Alice's Adventures in Wonderland
Lewis Carroll, 1865

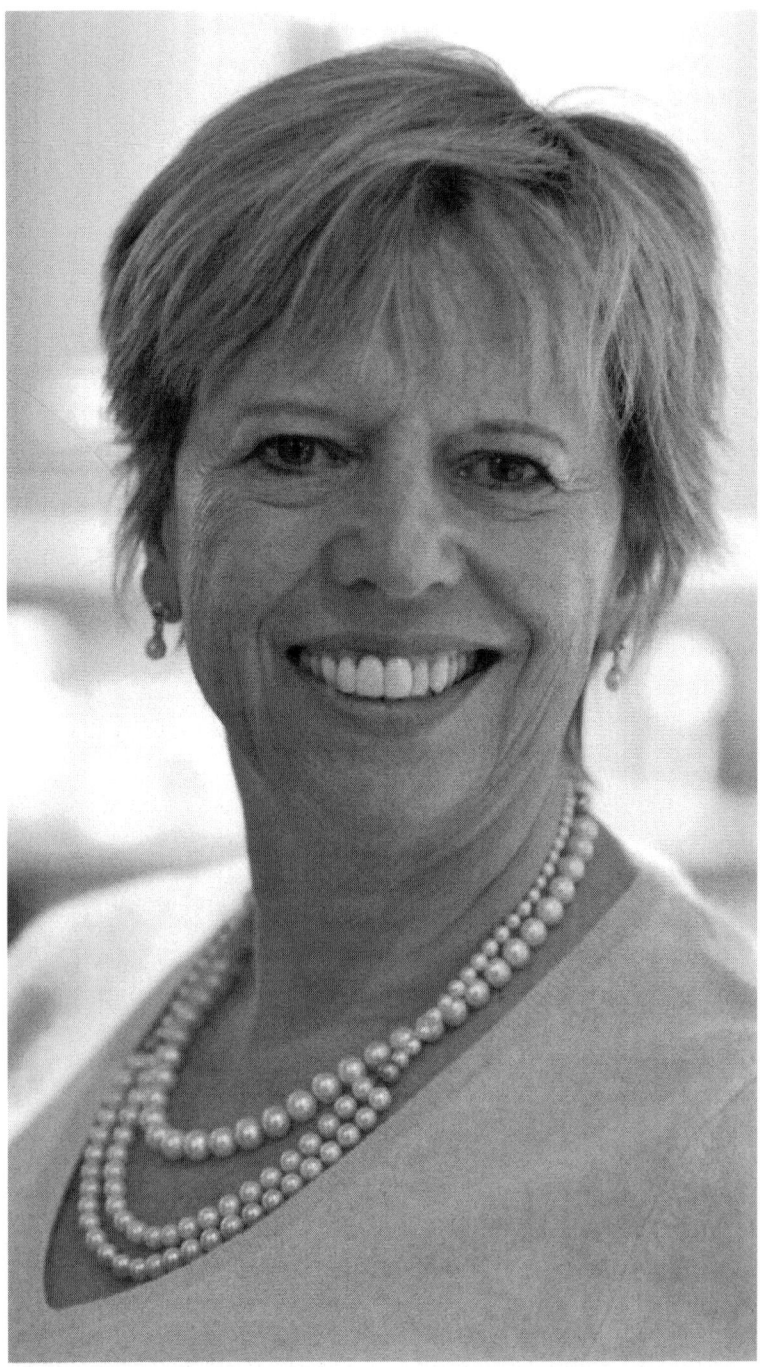

INTRODUCTION

"Why would anyone want to go and work in Qatar?" asked one of our friends.

"Because we've been headhunted," I said.

"OK" said another, "but why you, Penny? What do you know about the Middle East?"

Of course I knew nothing, but I also knew that it was my husband Lionel who they'd really been after. Retiring Rear Admiral, head of the Naval Medical Service … the options were out there and they had been keen to recruit him.

"Come and have lunch, Admiral," said the Savile Row-suited headhunter. From the safety of the oak-panelled dining room in a London club, he had extolled the virtues of life in the small Arab state of Qatar. "You'll love it. Good weather, your own pool, marble everywhere, very safe. No Arab Spring 'cos they don't need it."

Strong persuasion, but Lionel had remained unconvinced.

"Well, I'll think about it and discuss it with Penny,"

he'd said. "But you know she's also a doctor, a senior player in her hospital."

"No problem, have her send us her CV. They'll find her a job too."

Nothing to lose. I'd sent in my CV and we'd waited. In fact we had almost forgotten about it. We'd begun to talk about sailing the boat to distant lands and having a grown-up gap year or two.

Then the phone call had come.

"Lionel? They want Penny. Don't worry – they will find something for you as well."

A couple of visits to the Middle East and we were on: two job offers, both well paid, with a house included. After a summer sailing in home waters, we flew to Doha on 11 September 2012.

The boat was despatched to Turkish waters, so we could easily fly there and go sailing while on holiday, and our eldest son Jonathan and his wife, Anna, moved into our house in Hampshire while we headed off to this small Gulf state on a three-year contract.

Lionel had been there before as part of his military duties; indeed he had a wealth of experience of the region under the umbrella of Her Majesty's Armed Forces, but this was very different. We were going to be employed by the government of Qatar and the rules had changed. It quickly became evident that today's rules were opaque, inconsistent and difficult to follow. In spite of the skyscrapers, mobile phones and Land Cruisers speeding along four-lane highways through the desert, we soon felt we had gone back in time to the Middle Ages.

Settling into this new country with its wildly different culture from ours would not be easy and we realised that supporting each other and finding the humour in many situations would be vital. We knew people were literally *put on a plane* with no notice and we had no desire to end our employment so ignominiously.

This is the story of our time there. Did we cope? Yes – we did more than cope: we succeeded. It wasn't easy, but then adventures never are.

1

SHWAI SHWAI

Our plane starts its descent and I peer out. Blackness greets me beyond the window. And then scattered dots of light. Not cities, but what are they? Then it dawns on me: the bright spots I'm looking at are a representation of the huge wealth of this part of the world – oil fields. Lionel is the one to pick out the coastline, by more dots of light. We're flying over the Arabian Gulf – already we've been warned not to call it the Persian Gulf because Iran is not admired in these parts. We've been advised it's best not to upset Arab sensitivities, particularly when the Qatari government are now our paymasters. I begin once again to wonder why we have left our beautiful Hampshire farmhouse for the heat and dust of the desert.

And the answer? Easy – for the adventure! Who could resist being headhunted for a job with such a snappy title as Assistant Chief of Medical, Academic and Research Affairs? In truth, despite a series of interviews with Arabs and ex-pats, I have very little idea of exactly what the post entails. When it came to a job description, they have been irritatingly vague.

This is as much as I know. Hamad Medical

Corporation (HMC) is the government-sponsored health organisation; it could be loosely described as the Qatari equivalent of the British National Health Service. Named after the Emir himself, whose vision it is to build the best academic health enterprise in the Middle East, HMC employs twenty-two thousand people over eight hospitals and is growing by the day. New hospitals are being built and staff are being recruited from all over the world, particularly from the Arab regions and South East Asia. Within this large workforce there are nearly two thousand physicians. I will have responsibility for their professional development. Medicine is a constantly evolving discipline and training doesn't end with a degree. Learning continues throughout a doctor's career and I am the one who has to make this happen in Qatar.

Lionel, on the other hand, is to be Chief Executive and Medical Director of the fabulous new high-profile Heart Hospital, with fifteen hundred staff. He knows the Middle East, but for me it will be a new experience. Will they respect me or will I be brushed aside as a mere woman? How will I cope in this alien, male-dominated environment? I feel like the new girl at school.

The first day after landing in Qatar is a round of photos, form filling, applications for driving licences, medical examination, blood tests and meeting people, all of whom seem to be called Mohamed, Abdulla, Fatima or Amira. It is totally bewildering. We are chaperoned by a well-spoken, very proper English girl, Caroline, who helps us navigate this alien environment. She is charming but unfortunately has developed the Arab habit of only telling us what she perceives we need to know. Hence we become even more frustrated, Lionel in particular (he is very used to being in charge) as we feel we are being herded about with no control of our destiny.

Things come to a head when we are sent off to set up bank accounts. Abdul Aziz, a delightful Arab banker dressed in immaculate traditional robes with a carefully trimmed beard and twinkly eyes, ushers us into his office of the Qatar National Bank where we have been advised to apply for private banking arrangements. In Caroline's enthusiasm she has included another newly arrived ex-pat called Donald, in the same appointment and we all travel to the bank in a hospital car. Before we know it we are all in the office of the banker being asked about our personal financial circumstances. This is uncomfortable in the extreme, but our British reticence to make a fuss is trumped by our British discomfort to discuss personal matters publicly. We rebel and firmly tell Abdul that we are not all one family and what's more, we all want individual bank accounts. I certainly do not want a joint account: much as I trust my husband, I am used to and expect complete independence in financial matters. I subsequently discover this to be a wise decision.

We cannot be officially housed until all paperwork, most importantly, the Residence Permit, is complete, which means we are put up in one of the city's five-star hotels. We expect this will be for a week or so.

The hotel is built along grand lines. Everything is marble or covered in gold, giving an air of extreme opulence. There is a large central concourse with a domed glass ceiling across which hangs an enormous chandelier, measuring about ten feet across and twenty high. Beyond the chandelier the building rises about two hundred and fifty feet high, with the twenty-three floors positioned around a central void and their rooms arranged around the edge.

Coming out of my room I can lean over the balcony rail and look down eighteen vertiginous floors to the chandelier and concourse below. A pianist plays Palm Court music and Arab men and women sit sipping tea, eating cakes or smoking. There are a few westerners but these are more likely to be found in the bar, which is hidden away and can only be entered on production of identification. The locals are never there (or at least, not in traditional dress).

Outside there are fountains, discreet arbours where shisha pipes are smoked and gardens suffused with the heady smell of frangipani from the trees that grow interspersed with bougainvillea.

The lighting is magical and it is truly a delight to sip a glass of wine while gazing at the calm waters of the Arabian Gulf. We even try the shisha pipe. Our choice is rose flavoured and the hubble bubble is brought with great ceremony. Lighted coals are placed on the top and the *waiter* draws on the pipe before handing it to the guest. The cool smoke tastes like a mix of *pot pourri* and compost heap and makes us feel slightly heady. We subsequently discover that it does contain tobacco, but no other drugs. Once is enough.

There are eight public hospitals in Qatar under the auspices of Hamad Medical Corporation. They are a mix of exuberant architecture, state-of-the-art equipment and old-fashioned institutions more redolent of our old Victorian hospitals. The new builds have large central atria with beautiful courtyards and fountains, while the old ones have long corridors with flaky wall paint and chipped tiles. Lionel is fortunate to manage the newest hospital where the construction was personally overseen by the former Minister for Health, while my office in corporate headquarters is based in the old Women's Hospital. The new Women's Hospital is being built but we have no idea when it will open. Although I'm based in the Women's

Hospital, my work will take me to the others on campus and to three hospitals situated in different parts of the country.

Lionel's office sports an enormous highly polished desk trimmed with gold inlay, comfortable chairs and a table for conferences, all protected by an outer office where his secretary sits. Mine is small with rickety filing cabinets and a tiny coffee table that collapses if anyone perches on it. My secretary sits in a cubby-hole along the corridor. However, I am in the hub of the business and plenty of people pop in to see me as they pass by. This is crucial in an Arab society where relationships are so important if anything is to get done.

The working day is from 7am to 3pm and the rush-hour peak is around six-thirty. Ex-pats make a lot of fuss over driving in Qatar and some people simply don't bother, but use drivers instead. In truth it is not too bad but a thick skin is needed to cope with the constant blasting of horns. There are two basic rules: the driver to the left will cross in front of you and the driver to the right will also cross in front of you, so in essence wherever you are on one of the fast-flowing roundabouts, you can expect to be cut up. There is no lane discipline but for anyone who has ever driven a car in America, this is no great surprise. It is actually quite fun in a fairground dodgems sort of way, though nevertheless exhausting.

I become completely lost on one occasion. There are no meaningful signs, the road is a dual carriageway with nowhere to stop and my map is utterly useless. I feel like bursting into tears but what is the point? There is no one to help. *Pull yourself together*, I tell myself. So I keep driving randomly until suddenly I spy a familiar landmark. Then one of the hospitals miraculously appears. I am saved. Such a relief and then a feeling of, "Yes I can cope. I can do this." From then on, my innate curiosity mingled with determination becomes my foremost emotion.

I have my photograph taken so the hospital can send out a press release. It appears in the Arab press: the managing director is flanked by her two Qatari deputy chiefs. Her three western ones, including me, are shown in slightly smaller frames, no doubt denoting our status (same job, but not Qatari). One is an eminent Swedish professor who, among his many achievements, sat on the committee for allocation of Nobel prizes. He is amazingly self-effacing and seems genuinely interested in my prosaic career. We chat and get on well, but no sooner is the press release issued than the Swede gives up and returns home. I never really find out why. The other westerner is moved to the job that he had initially been promised, so I find myself as the only westerner – and the only female – working alongside two Arab men. How is this going to work? I plan to observe and try to keep quiet.

In this traditional society, women's roles tend to be based around the home and family, yet there are notable exceptions such as our own managing director. She is a relatively young woman who is well educated and has achieved meteoric promotion. I have yet to meet her and am intrigued to see how our relationship might develop. Somewhat naively I suppose that, as the most senior woman in the organisation after her, I might develop a bond with her and share some common understanding of success within a man's world. The reality turns out to be much less cosy.

I request a meeting with her. In my world this would be a courtesy and I expect to do the running rather than be summoned. Her British secretary responds with a request for an agenda. *Fair enough* I think, although it seems a bit excessive for a joining meeting. So I duly comply and am given a date. Which is cancelled. A new time is proposed and so it goes on – cancellations and postponements until it becomes clear that I am never going to meet this woman one-to-one.

In truth, I'm not alone. Visiting foreign dignitaries find the same problem. Meetings are cancelled and reinstated at short notice: it is all part of the Arab version of timeliness. It happens at board meetings too. No one turns up on time, then the ones who have arrived drift off and need summoning back. So it goes on that a meeting scheduled for an hour might take ninety minutes, of which only forty are fruitful discussion.

The Arabs love employing external advisors, so there are numerous management consultants from various countries around the world, especially the USA, Canada and the UK. In my first couple of weeks, there is a presentation given by a British-based company. I am invited to attend and assess them.

"Sit here, on the boss's right hand," advises one of the chiefs.

"Really?" I say, not wishing to be too pushy.

"Of course – you are the new girl. Sit there, next to her."

So I do. The MD swans in, abaya flowing, and the presentation began. Questions ensue and I ask a pertinent one, or so I think. She turns to me. At last, I presume, she's worked me out and we can move on. Wrong!

"And who are you?" is her response to my pithy interrogation. What abject embarrassment for me and intense irritation that no one had seen fit to make introductions properly at the beginning of the meeting. Luckily my response is met with a smile and an apology to cover her own embarrassment. Once she realises who I am she says, "I look forward to meeting you properly."

It makes me reflect that in spite of the national press coverage, the announcements in the hospital, and the warm welcome there might be people who are less keen on a Western woman doctor and do not wish me to succeed.

I decide to ask some questions. Calling on the director of finance is not difficult as his office is next to mine (when I am finally given an office).

"You have some very good people working in this organisation," I say, "so I don't understand why you employ so many outside agencies."

That strikes a nerve. "There are too many," he responds. "They don't understand us. They cost too much. They should go."

So there are definite tensions. The finance director is one of the traditionalists who is less keen on outside intervention, although he was educated in the States. He is also highly moral and is dismayed at the number of western agencies trying to make money out of the Qatari wealth. He has a good point.

I realise that if I am to succeed then I must understand the Arab mentality and my plan of learning their ways and proceeding gently is a good one. *Shwai shwai* as they say in Arabic, slowly, slowly.

The first week in any new job is emotionally draining and this is no exception. I have spent the week at one formal meeting (to which the secretariat irritatingly forgot to invite me, so I had to make a small fuss) and lots of individual meetings with key members of staff. I have gone to meet them on their own territory, which seems to be appreciated, though I wonder how my exuberant personality will be perceived in this collective culture where individualism is less highly respected than in the West.

The first challenge is whether to shake hands. Some

Qatari men refuse to shake hands with a woman, but the more culturally aware of these will signify by putting his right hand to his chest and bowing. I quickly learn not to extend my hand until theirs is proffered. Conversation is initially very general with much talk about family, visits to England, and medicine in general as a profession: I have been warned that I might need several meetings before getting onto the business in hand.

There's a project plan for me to follow, with a main action committee supported by several sub-committees. Perusing the papers from these various committees, however, several things become apparent: the terms of reference keep changing, no one can decide who is the chair, the next meeting is not arranged and there are no action points in the minutes.

Nothing has happened over the summer because of Ramadan and holidays, so the accompanying Gantt chart – designed to plot progress against targets – is a complete fiction. The cynic might say that this is not dissimilar to the situation in the NHS and I confess that I am not unduly concerned because in spite of the cultural differences I still believe that I will change things.

Simple decisions like what to wear become important: I'm acutely aware of sensibilities and choose my clothes carefully for work. Knees and elbows should be covered and necklines should be very modest, so my lovely Italian dresses which would be perfect in this climate are entirely unsuitable. Air-conditioning is kept fiercely cold so a jacket or similar is necessary indoors.

Most of the indigenous women are dressed in the long black abaya, a robe-like dress accompanied by a scarf (*shayla*) that covers their hair. They glide along looking surprisingly elegant, particularly since they are all wearing expensive killer heels and carrying designer handbags.

Some show their faces, often very beautiful with heavily made-up eyes, while others cover their faces completely, which is disconcerting and slightly spooky.

Doha is a cosmopolitan society. Western women in the hotels dress freely, and the Muslim women from other countries who merely cover their hair with coloured scarves look independent and modern. The men are dressed in traditional white robes and head-dress, but at the swimming pool they wear western casual clothes.

At the hotel we see an extraordinary sight; a young family with the man in shorts, T-shirt and baseball cap, little girls in sweet polka-dot dresses and their mother completely covered from head to toe in black. I've already learned that there is a problem with vitamin D deficiency among the population generally but especially in the women.

I am finding it unnerving to see these apparently faceless women walking around but when in the Ladies yesterday, failing at washing my hands because I couldn't work the taps, a woman threw back her veil to help me; she was young, smiled and we had a good non-spoken conversation.

At work, I am repeatedly told about the strong tribal ties in this region and the off-stage decisions that are made. Influence comes through the *majilis,* which are gatherings of the men in a family. Many are related to the Royal family and are therefore only a phone call away from the Emir. This makes any organisational structure difficult to maintain and also difficult to develop. It becomes a constant theme.

There is a learned helplessness exhibited by many of the staff – Arabs and other races alike. I am not an office worker by profession but even I could see that the filing system in the department was archaic, chaotic and plainly did not work. There were piles of papers scattered about the floor, which had to be navigated through in order to reach anyone's desk.

"We need an electronic system, as paperless as possible," I suggest.

"Oh yes, you are right," replies Theresa, the Filipina office supervisor. "We have been saying that for years".

"Great. So what have you done?"

"Well nothing. We are waiting for someone to tell us what we need."

"But you know your systems. Can't you put some ideas together?" I ask.

The answer is no. Self-determination as a concept is not an option.

Finance for big projects is not difficult to find, but minor bureaucracies abound and the rules of engagement are still very opaque. The city with its magnificent new buildings still feels like a frontier town on the edge of the desert. There are building works everywhere in the hospitals with some beautiful new courtyards under construction for the patients. Those that have been finished have fountains, flowers, and an atmosphere of peace and tranquillity.

However, people are very reluctant to go outside and I am constantly being offered cars to take me two hundred yards because of the heat, which – they say – is impossible to walk in. Or maybe people just don't like walking. I do walk and they find me eccentric. They also worry that the air-conditioning in my office is not working because I refuse to walk into a cold blast from the intense heat outside. I keep it at a gentle level.

Small things tax my concentration, such as the fact that the calendar facility on Microsoft Outlook shows a working week from Monday to Friday and I am forced to fiddle around to make it read Sunday to Thursday. Even so, Monday feels like Tuesday and so on. The day is punctuated by the call to prayer and it is important when meeting people around midday that their need to pray is respected. They will not terminate the conversation, out of politeness, but will be uncomfortable.

I seem to be spending every second of the day observing, trying to understand and make sense of this new world.

Walking through the long hospital corridors, I am constantly greeted by strangers on the hospital staff with a respectful "Good morning" or even "Good morning, madam", but these workers tend to be Filipino or Indian in origin. The traditionally dressed Arabs of either gender do not greet me and I confess to being wary of making eye contact, because of cultural sensitivities.

Living in five-star luxury sounds grand but can never be home. The food is excellent and the staff are charming, but we are keen to have our own place. The good news is that we've made progress on getting our Residence Permit. This is important for several reasons: it means that we can live independently, we can have debit and credit cards, we can get a licence to buy alcohol (and bacon, it is rumoured) but most importantly we will get our passports back with multi-exit visas.

It is a very benign society but nevertheless there are restrictions such as needing permission to leave the country, unless you do something wrong, in which case you can be thrown out within twenty-four hours.

The weekend is very welcome and we are off to brunch in the hotel. We discover, when we turn up in shorts and T-shirts, that this is the social occasion of the week for ex-pats and is an opportunity for (amongst other delicacies) traditional Sunday lunch with a roast, Yorkshire pudding and all the trimmings, but also an excuse to dress up. The Western women are in high heels and silk dresses, the men in smart casual. We sneak off and change before reappearing in appropriate garb.

2

LEARNING THE ROPES

e decide that we really should learn a few words or phrases of Arabic. At Lionel's Heart Hospital, only four of the fifteen-hundred staff are Westerners, so he really is in a foreign land. We investigate the possibility of lessons and his secretary Noora, who has *wasta*, is on the case. *Wasta* simply means that you know how to influence and get things done around here. This may be because you are from a prominent family or may simply be that you know everyone.

It is a fine example of a mixture of tacit knowledge, nepotism and good old-fashioned charm, to the right people of course. Noora has all of this and proudly announces that she has found us a brilliant teacher, a professor of Arabic at the university and we are honoured because he doesn't usually teach Arabic to people like us.

"How did you manage it?" we demand.

"The professor is my father," she says with a wry smile.

We've no choice but to follow her through the chaotic

evening traffic to his house. The noise of the road has gone and we find ourselves outside a splendid villa with a lemon grove adjacent to it. There she leads us through a gate in a high wall, to a haven of peace beyond.

We're ushered into the house by a bevy of Filipina maids and the professor's wife. Coffee and cakes are served before the great man makes his entrance. Although we are not hungry it would be rude to refuse the fig roll cakes, which are filled with crushed rose petals, fragrant and delicious.

Lionel has already picked up a few words of Arabic from his drivers and is convinced we should not attempt to understand the writing but simply learn a few expressions with the correct pronunciation. So imagine our dismay when the professor sits between us at his dining table and proceeds to teach us to write the Arabic alphabet. At the same time he pronounces the letters and encourages us to speak. Unfortunately many of the letters sound the same, essentially a noise in the back of the throat that to the untutored ear sounds like someone attempting to be sick.

Well, we try. We make our dismal vomiting sounds, all of which are wrong, but at least we can copy the letters. Except that he isn't happy with those either. We are, of course, writing from right to left and, because he is a classical Arabic scholar, he insists on showing us three different notations for each letter. I confess that I don't understand but it is something about the name of the letter, its pronunciation and the way it is written within a word or sentence. He races through the letters and although Lionel is manfully keeping up, he loses me completely.

The experience is truly humiliating, akin to being a remedial child in kindergarten. Our next lesson is fixed and we dutifully do our homework, learning the letters as instructed and he tests us at the beginning of the session.

We don't do too badly but we still haven't finished the alphabet so the first session's process is repeated. We are both tired at the end of the day, the traffic has been dreadful on the journey there and although the professor is very kind, especially when he sees that I am close to tears with frustration, it is all too much.

We both realise that we were being overambitious so we manage to extricate ourselves from the arrangement without any loss of face on his part. In truth, we suspect he didn't really want to teach us anyway and it is probably a relief to him also.

However, we did feel honoured to be allowed this fascinating glimpse into an Arab home. The rooms are large, with huge chandeliers, marble floors, heavy curtains and gold embellishments everywhere. I am reminded of extravagantly decorated baroque churches.

As we leave, his wife beckons to us.

"Come and see the garden," she says.

We follow her into the warm night air where the scent from the lemon grove is intoxicating.

"The scent of those lemons is amazing," I remark, whereupon she summons one of the maids.

"Pick a lemon for our guest," she says, brusquely.

It's an interesting culture where no one is expected to do anything for themselves if there is someone else available. During our lesson, Lionel had taken off his jacket so the professor assumed he was too hot and summoned a maid to turn up the air-conditioning. This onerous task involves pressing a button but would be far beneath the master of the household.

Things are no different in the hospital. Lionel has an Italian coffee machine in his office but an Arab guest looked up in horror, quite unable to cope when Lionel leapt out of his chair to make the coffee.

"Please, Dr Lionel," he said, "sit and talk to me and get someone else to do that."

When Arabic coffee is served, the ritual is to take a small half cup which is replenished by holding out the cup for more and when one has had enough then the cup is shaken from side to side. Incidentally, this Arab beverage does not taste of coffee but is delicious with a mix of spices, cardamom being the most prominent (unlike NHS coffee, which doesn't taste of anything at all). Of course this ritual presumes that there is someone to stand in the corner of the room just in case anyone wants more coffee, while the conversation goes on around him.

We make a similar observation when we wander into an upholstery shop in the souq, where an elderly toothless Arab is sitting on a large cushion, talking on his mobile phone while an Indian man is squatting on the floor, busily reupholstering a chair. He looks like a skilled craftsman but he is summoned to go and find fabric swatches for us while the Arab owner chats to us in completely unintelligible broken English. Needless to say, we decide against trading with him, partly because he has no suitable fabric but also because communication would be impossible.

Because we need to travel around independently, we each hire a car. Lionel is worried for my safety and I've promised to behave myself. Road rage is a universal phenomenon, especially here where the men drive their cars as if they were riding camels – hard, fast and randomly. Driving in my rented car, I am hooted at by someone on my tail in the middle lane. There is nowhere to go but when it is safe I pull over into the inner lane whereupon he proceeds to cut in front of me.

Shaking my head and laughing at this appalling driving, I then realise that my response has been noticed by the bad driver who gesticulates wildly at me before turning off right in front of me. *Idiot*, I think (and other less polite expressions) but I am still laughing at the absurdity when he does a quick U-turn and drives at me at great speed before swerving away at the last minute.

No points for guessing that he is an Arab in full robes and head-dress driving a huge four-wheel-drive Land Cruiser complete with go-faster stripes. Lionel suggests, "I should think being laughed at by a western woman in a poxy little car was an affront to his manhood."

Later, when in traffic today, the driver of a car in front opens his door and spits onto the road – a good footballer's gob – I suppress my expression of disgust. It would seem that a serene expression is safest. Maybe that's really why the women veil — so they can express their emotions with impunity.

But what about the working environment? For me, one of the best things about being a doctor is the patients. They keep me grounded and remind me why I embarked on this profession. However, I also realise that without good clinical systems, we fail to do the best for our patients. For example, I might suspect that a breast lump in a patient is cancerous but if I cannot do an ultrasound, take a biopsy and get the result to her quickly, then her life will be dreadful for a few weeks, whatever the outcome. Patients always say to me, "The waiting is the worst bit".

My job in the UK was a combination of hands-on doctor, clinical leader/manager and educator. I would have relished the opportunity to treat patients in the multi-cultural setting of Qatar, but I am appointed to run the show. People ask me if I would do some clinics, report some CT scans, do some biopsies; but I decline. Why? It's such a wrench to give up seeing patients and yet it is the right thing. I reason that if I have to be called to a meeting at short notice I'll be expected to attend. Fine, but if I have a clinic then for me the patients would always come first. Would this be a conflict and would my new Qatari masters understand my viewpoint? I elect to give up direct patient contact. It is the right move.

I have to adjust to my new role in an alien environment. I know that being a doctor gives me kudos but I feel the need to use that advantage carefully lest I am judged as a mere administrator. As ever, *shwai, shwai,* slowly, slowly is my tactic.

This is how I started: without a clinical role it would be difficult to understand the hospital, so I have taken to wandering around the corridors just to get a feel for the place. It is very multicultural with different nationalities, languages, dress and very few Westerners among this mix. Certain nationalities appear to be assigned to particular staff groups. For example, my secretary, the wonderfully named Honeylet, is from the Philippines as are many of the secretarial staff and I hear them talking in their local tongue.

One of the senior secretaries in my patch, Abdulrahman, is Sudanese and he is very supportive of me, taking me personally to meet various awkward people such as the transport manager. Male secretaries and male clerical staff are common out here. They are usually from one of the Asian nations, never from Qatar and only rarely from Arab nations such as Sudan. It was the transport manager who approved my (very beaten-up) temporary loan car and he likes to see prospective drivers personally. He made no secret of the fact that he dislikes foreigners and embarked on a conversation on the Holy Book, the Holy Month and why fasting is important, before launching into a long diatribe against colonialism.

He did manage to concede that as far as colonial masters went, the British were marginally better than the

French, whereupon Abdulrahman replied staunchly that frankly his country wanted the British back to sort everything out. I was excluded from the conversation at this point until Tricky Transport Man turned to Abdulrahman and asked, referring to me, "So, can this doctor drive?"

I must have somehow passed muster because I was taken to my car personally by Tricky Transport Man, whereupon we both examined the car for bumps and scratches before I drove it away. It is an accepted fact that the bodywork on most cars will be less than pristine.

There are flower and chocolate shops in the hospitals. These are set out as stalls in the large concourses and sell extravagant displays of flowers, particularly in the maternity wing, where huge gifts of chocolates are also sold. These may be several feet high, with elaborate mosaics of foil-covered chocolates, mounted among glorious flowers. It is all rather wonderful if completely over the top.

A western friend observes that her aesthetic has been somewhat altered since living here and she finds herself looking at objects and thinking, "That needs a little gold rim!"

The hospital corridors and public areas are busy with white-coated doctors sweeping along in ward rounds, nurses wearing surgical scrubs and workmen – usually Indian – in blue overalls. Last Thursday in the afternoon I suddenly encountered dozens of workers clad in grey uniforms embroidered with the legend *Domestic Staff,* the women wearing identical headscarves tied at the back of the head. The women were talking animatedly in a language that sounded a little like Chinese: they looked Asian but I couldn't pin their nationality down further. The men were a different race and judging from my conversations with the hotel domestic staff, I think they were Bangladeshi. There were literally hundreds of these people all moving towards a destination at the back of the hospital.

As I turned corners, there were more of these grey-clad workers spilling out of every doorway. I still haven't quite worked it all out, but possibly they were going to collect their wages at the end of the week before being bused home. I still don't know where the women come from. These migrant workers, including many nursing staff, are very poorly paid and viewed with disdain by the locals.

Wages might be low yet are much better than those in their home countries. When I arrived at work on Sunday, I was told that Honeylet had gone back to the Philippines because of a family matter, but no one knew for how long. Relating this to a colleague, the immediate response was, "So she's been deported".

Who knows?

When I need to visit the hospital in the north, about an hour's drive away, I am not keen to drive myself across the desert so, following guidance, I request a car. However, I'm informed that because I have been lent a car by the corporation, I must use *it* for this journey, though a driver will be provided. This is duly arranged, memos sent (the memo is an important bit of organisational currency) and on Sunday morning, Yasser (tea-boy, stationery dispenser and general gofer) takes me over to Transport. There are several men milling about outside the offices, which resemble a concrete cell block, and while Yasser negotiates in Arabic, I hang about outdoors as I am not invited in out of the sun and heat.

They claim to know nothing but eventually a driver is found for me and we go to my loan car, having assured them that it is full of petrol. My driver is straight out of

Lawrence of Arabia with long flowing robes, head-dress with tassels down his back, worry beads, bad teeth and an aroma which is a mixture of male sweat and Arabian perfume. He speaks no English and off we go.

At this juncture, forget David Lean films with vistas of romantic sand dunes and dashing Arab princes riding their thoroughbred stallions over horizons. This landscape is completely flat, very dusty and there is the occasional dead bush. There is nothing else apart from the occasional building site, but at least the road is good and inevitably we drive very fast. Eventually we encounter some habitation and my driver turns to me gesticulating wildly, clearly asking me where to go. I have no idea and nor does he.

We turn into a small health centre and he stops the car, so I tell him to wait. I go in, where I find a man in a white coat with a label saying 'Doctor'. He is charming, speaks English and happily responds to my request to speak to my driver in Arabic. It takes about five minutes of intensive voluble chat – plus gesticulations – to tell him to turn right, then straight on until we reach the hospital. Having arrived there, we stop somewhat randomly outside the Haemodialysis Unit, so once again, in I go and find a very helpful pharmacist and an Indian porter who offers to take me through the hospital to the office of the Medical Director.

This strikes me as a dangerous ploy since I may never see my car and driver again, so I herd porter and driver, who has by now appeared, and insist that the porter comes in the car with us to the main reception. Amazingly I am on time for my appointment and am treated like a queen. It is a good meeting, with coffee and a tour of the hospital, including an explanation of the isolation rooms designated for infectious diseases.

Before coming here, Lionel and I had to provide a

certificate stating that we had never had tuberculosis, yet there is a high incidence of TB in the migrant workers working in the industrial city in the north. They come mainly from the Indian sub-continent, without their families and are housed in dormitory-like accommodation. They work in this industrial city that covers over thirty square kilometres and is a conglomeration of refinery, tanker port and pipelines. It abuts the huge natural gas field which projects out into the Gulf towards Iran. Unless I had looked it up on the internet I would have never known of its existence, yet it is the source of the country's wealth. To be fair, I am new here so I do not presume any conspiracy or cover-up.

The episode with the enraged Arab driver made me realise that a decent car is a necessity. Given the state of the driving, traffic and roads, it is clearly important that we have our own cars which are well built, safe and with reliable acceleration in order to get out of trouble. I choose a good European make, a Volvo four-wheel drive and Lionel goes for an American tank, namely a 5.3 litre Chevrolet Tahoe.

I choose the lease-purchase option and he elects to take a personal bank loan (because only then would we be allowed, inexplicably, to take the car out of the country, should we feel the need to escape across the desert). It all sounds astoundingly simple – if only.

For the deposit on the car, which has to be in cash, I have to transfer some money from the UK. So, trotting off to the garage with my thirty thousand riyals (about five thousand pounds), I count it out and expect to drive the car away. Wrong. This is the first process in registering the car and so it goes on, with trips back and forth until eventually I can drive my new Volvo away … except it isn't exactly my car. I am still waiting for a resident's permit, so the garage helpfully arrange for it to be in their name in the interim. It is all very simple.

"You just have to sign a paper in Arabic then you can have the car," says my Egyptian car salesman.

Frankly by this stage I would have signed anything but Lionel is more cautious.

"Well, OK," he responds, "But at least can we see my wife's name at the top of the document?"

Carefully my salesman places his pen at the top right hand side of the document.

"But of course," he says and, you've guessed it, writes something completely unintelligible in Arabic.

Well it all works out in the end, but not before I pledge the hire purchase payments, not with a direct debit but by writing twenty-two post-dated personal cheques, which I leave in the custody of the garage to cash at monthly intervals.

What about Lionel? His salesman is a pale, skinny Lebanese girl with fiercely plucked and painted eyebrows. Her hair is scraped back in a Croydon facelift and the answer to any question is, "Yes, of course," delivered in the abrasive clipped tones worthy of any Bond villain.

"Can I drive my car away tomorrow?" Lionel asks.

And the answer is, "Yes, of course."

This is pure fiction and he goes through similar convoluted procedures as I have, even though he has waited for his Residence Permit. There were some good things, such as the personal bank loan that was granted, no question, that very day. The money was simply transferred into his account. However when he suggests transferring it over to the garage's account (same bank) this suggestion is met with astonishment.

No, cash is preferred. So off he goes across town with roughly forty thousand pounds in Qatari Riyals in a brown paper bag. On arrival at the garage they calmly put it through their on-site cash counter and all is well.

"Yes, of course," is only one of several stock answers to any query. Others include, "No problem" and "In the next five minutes."

In fact, any answer but "No" is given. How to judge the truth? Depending on the ethnicity of the person, there are often some non-verbal clues, the commonest being a barely perceptible head motion that manages to be simultaneously a nod and a shake, culminating in a subtle figure of eight. The more vigorous the movement, the more likely that he is talking complete bullshit. But most importantly, I learn to watch the eyes. Dodgy and evasive translates as "not a hope in hell," despite the promise of "yes, sir, immediately!"

I fill up my new Volvo with petrol for the princely sum of thirty-two-and-a half-riyals, which is about six quid. The guide books recommend rounding up the bill in order to give the petrol pump attendant a tip, so I give him thirty-five riyals and with great largesse tell him to keep the change. He gives me a strange look and points out that the QR5 note is in fact a QR500 note – and I was priding myself on being able to read numbers written in Arabic script. Of course, had I turned the note over, it was all written in English anyway!

My new office is in the corporate headquarters, but I am more comfortable in the hospital, having worked in them all my adult life. It is an interesting observation that many patients and their relatives instinctively dislike and distrust hospitals whereas healthcare workers are completely at ease there, a fact worth remembering when patients and their families are anxious or even angry. They are simply scared stiff.

Throughout all the HMC hospitals are signs in English

and Arabic and one of the most notable reproduced below, advises relatives how to behave when visiting patients.
Etiquette of visiting patient (published by the Religious guidance and Da'wa department):

- ☐ *Select a suitable time for the visit*
- ☐ *Avoid staying with the patient for a long time*
- ☐ *Respect patient's condition, do not raise your voice in his presence and do not disclose information which would upset him*
- ☐ *Pray for the patient sincerely*
- ☐ *Console the patient using an optimistic approach and give hope of recovery*
- ☐ *Remind the patient about the rewards of patience*
- ☐ *Do not make the patient doubtful regarding the doctor or the treatment plan*
- ☐ *Avoid mentioning non-suitable suggestions to the patient*

Imagine such exhortations in a British hospital! I did hear people volunteering to pray for patients when I was in America, but we British tend to be much more subtle regarding religious matters and even the chaplains do their praying discreetly. The sub-text of protecting the patient from unwelcome news is interesting and very much part of the culture here.

Relatives will go to great lengths to keep a diagnosis of cancer from the patient and I hear of one case where a daughter was proud that even on his deathbed, her father thought he was suffering from anaemia, not the prostate cancer that finally killed him. It would seem that openness is not embraced as a concept and questioning the doctor appears to be actively discouraged. Yet complaints are numerous and patients and their families demanding.

Expectations are high, but there are few attempts to manage them. An out-patient booking system has recently been installed, which is having some effect. Previously patients would simply turn up and demand to see the doctor of their choice, usually because they had seen that particular doctor before or because there was a family connection. If you are not from a local family then the Emergency Department is the only place, as there are very few GP surgeries.

Relatives from local Qatari families are unwilling to take their turn in the Emergency Department and stories abound of doctors being physically dragged away from treating a migrant worker in order to see a local patient first. This has resulted in a kind of local apartheid where Qataris are treated in separate bays, in order to diminish the acts of violence and aggression. And I thought the Emergency Department on a Saturday night in Portsmouth was bad.

Yet overall, people are generally warm and friendly. I make formal appointments to see prominent Arab doctors in order to discuss policy and strategy and am made very welcome. I'm given their delicious Arabic coffee, flavoured with cardamom and saffron and I'm offered sticky pastries with chopped pistachios or occasionally fresh dates, which look revolting yet taste sublime. There is much small talk and people are amazed when I say that we had a good laugh. I may not be getting the business done but at least we can share a joke and I suspect this relationship-building is crucial.

It is particularly important as a westerner to show that you have some understanding of these cultural mores. An abrasive *let's get straight down to business* approach does not work in the Arab world.

Exactly how well I am doing is hard to judge. Lionel,

needless to say, is flying in those terms but he needs to be. The prestigious new Heart Hospital has no governance, failing leadership and a need to meet external regulation. The place is in relationship meltdown with various warring factions, interventions by the Royal family and an expectation that Lionel will sort it out. Never frightened of confronting the issues, he asks directly whether a consultant attended his out-patient clinic and the reply is strongly affirmative, whereas the out-patient manager is perfectly clear that the consultant has seen no one in out-patients for months, but leaves it up to his junior staff.

Meanwhile there are votes of no confidence, disreputable memos signed by members of the same family discrediting other staff members, and only this week, Lionel has had several grown men and women in tears in his office.

Nevertheless the standard of clinical practice here can be high. I attend a Mortality and Morbidity meeting in the Heart Hospital where two cases are discussed in detail. The debate is scholarly and heated at times but there are some very wise voices among the assembled senior clinicians.

I experience the same commitment to good medical practice at a Grand Round in the education centre. These usually take the format of a junior doctor presenting a recent interesting case followed by a discussion about the treatment plans, the outcomes and how this all fits with the recent academic literature. It is a good forum for the juniors to hone their public speaking skills and for the senior doctors to guide (and in some cases to show off) their knowledge. Everyone learns so ultimately the patients also benefit.

There is a pecking order among the staff. Lionel's senior physician (and former minister of health) chairs the proceedings, asks the pithy questions and when he alone has decided that the meeting is over (regardless of any guidance on the timetable), he announces that the meeting is closed … then sweeps out with a flamboyant swish of his robes. There is no question of a cosy chat afterwards.

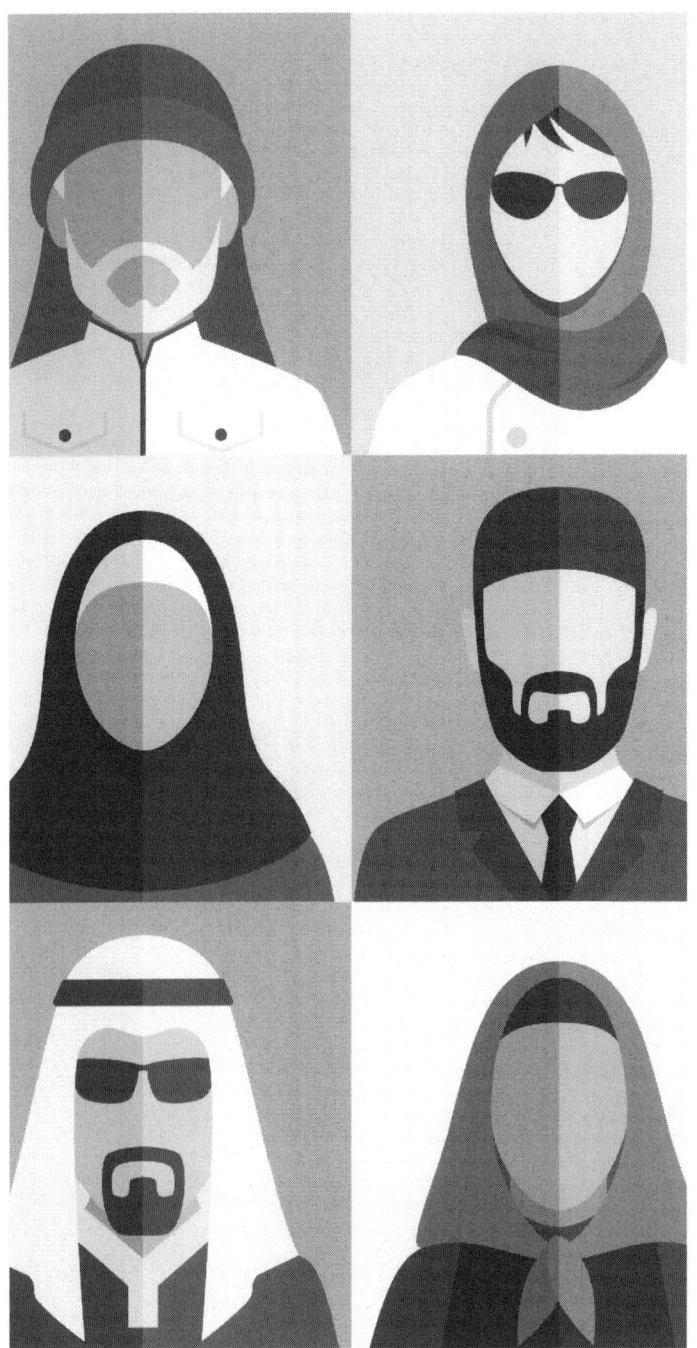

3

HOT BUT NOT BOTHERED

I t's difficult to believe that this is just the annual hospital awards beano. The venue is massive, shaped like an enormous tent with a high central dome, a stage at one edge and seating for eight hundred people around white linen-draped tables, each seating ten. The VVIPs with gold tickets are in the front two rows of tables, the VIPs slightly further back and the rest take their chances. The whole place is bathed in a silvery light with lasers flashing across the room and stilt dancers, clad in fantastic white glittering costumes, parade around. A dancer in a bubble moves around the tables and the whole scene is reminiscent of a winter wonderland. The temperature outside is thirty-seven degrees Celsius, but inside the air conditioning is working overtime.

We are treated to an amazing light show depicting images of the hospital as it seemingly emerged from the desert and our guide for this is an eagle who appears to be flying with us. Beautiful and extravagantly done, though the ensuing awards are somewhat lacklustre. Maybe such things always are, but it occurred to us that some champagne would have fizzed up the proceedings more than lemonade or mango juice.

Traditional sword dancers bumble around on the stage accompanied by drummers. Swords are being waved about with abandon and not for the first time, it occurs to us that ensuring our necks are well out of the way of such dancing was a judicious plan.

Frothy and superficial with entertainment galore for the glitterati – but where are the ordinary workers? Have they been invited to this extravaganza? Sadly no. A few representatives from the winning teams are hauled onto the stage from their tables at the back of the room. Most of the hospital staff can only dream about attending such an event.

Meanwhile there is day-to-day work to do. And it all seems very normal. There is a chairman, a secretary taking minutes, an agenda and the usual accompanying paperwork. We sit around the boardroom table and the meeting starts. Anarchy could not begin to describe the ensuing scene. Admittedly people stay in their chairs but the dialogue is vivid, people talk across each other, the chairman is completely ineffectual and at one stage I spot the lawyer adjacent to me reading his papers backwards, because they are, not unreasonably, in Arabic.

The problem starts when he quotes from those papers (in English) provoking a vociferous challenge from another Arab. "Read it in Arabic," he demands, "then we will translate", the sub-text being that he clearly does not trust his lawyer colleague.

The body language is florid, with hands waving, worry beads jangling and the men constantly fiddling with their headgear. The *ghuttra* is the long flowing white, or red-and-white chequered, headdress which is held in place by a black *aghal* or rope ring. There are numerous ways to wear this and the most traditional is in the style of little boys playing shepherds in the school nativity play.

However there are many alternative styles with asymmetric coiling of the *ghuttra*, with maybe one edge hanging nonchalantly over a shoulder; sometimes the *aghal* rope is covered by multiple pleats and the men constantly fiddle, in the manner of teenage girls tossing their flowing hair, as they readjust their look.

Overall the look is so uniform that individuality is reached through such variations plus differences in beards and cufflinks. A friend who teaches English to young Qatari men reveals that their conversation revolves around three Cs: cars, camels and cufflinks.

The meeting ends in disarray as everyone simply stands and leaves and the poor Filipina secretary has no idea what to record. Frankly, I cannot help. I confess that I probably added to the confusion, by also talking at loud volume and waving my arms around. It is the only way to get a point across, even if there are no decisions ultimately made. Maybe I am settling in more than I realise.

It might be expected that relocating to a new country would involve a certain amount of personal admin and although it seems excessive here, we have to keep reminding ourselves that foreigners moving to Britain might share our sentiments. The first hurdle is the Residence Permit, without which nothing can happen. We are fortunate because we receive this within four weeks along with a multi-exit visa, as hoped for.

This latter piece of documentation is particularly important as without it, permission needs to be sought from your employer for every trip out of the country. Also, should we go abroad without our Residence Permit then on our return it would mean starting the whole process again from scratch, assuming we *were* let back in.

The other perk granted to us as senior people in the organisation is that we are allowed to take holiday within ten months of starting work. A basic grade nurse, say from India or the Philippines, is not even allowed to leave the country within the first ten months.

Lionel, in his role as chief executive, is phoned at night by an immigration official to check that he approves one of his staff going home to visit a sick relative. Imagine the trepidation of a staff member waiting at the airport wondering whether she will be blocked from getting on the plane unless this has been clarified.

We assume the Residence Permit is a mere formality but subsequently understand that it is only granted after intense scrutiny by the Criminal Investigation Department branch of the Ministry of Interior. This varies depending on nationality. As Brits, it probably is cursory but for others, especially Shia Muslims from neighbouring states, it can take months. Qatar, like its neighbour Saudi Arabia, practises the strict Wahhabi form of Sunni Islam. Thankfully, the legal system and punitive methods are much more lenient: there are no beheadings and mutilations here.

A mobile phone is very necessary and we purchased ours on the first day. All business is done on it, including banking which is excellent (in spite of the shaky start), with text messages arriving instantly after every transaction. This can be galling for a wife if she shares a joint account with her husband as every purchase she makes is immediately communicated to the husband via his mobile phone. I am very relieved that we decided against joint accounts, though I am amused to learn that Lionel has been given an extra credit card.

"What is this for?" he enquires.

"For your wife, of course," comes the reply.

Interestingly, I am not given an extra one for him. We receive a very personal service from our bank manager who even comes to our hotel one evening to get a signature, but only because things haven't gone smoothly, for unexplained reasons. The rule of three here means that if you get a result within the first three attempts that is considered a stunning success.

Curiously, the coyly named Distribution Centre is the place for buying booze and in order to do so it is necessary to have a less coyly named Liquor Permit (a permit to drink alcohol, and therefore also to buy it). The amount spent per month on alcohol is strictly controlled and is related to salary, so the better paid are allowed to drink more, or so we're told. We're both allowed permits and the clerk who processes mine exercises inordinate care over taking my photograph. At last he is happy as he presents me with the permit. My image is appalling. I look like I need to be in rehab. It is enough to drive me to drink – perhaps they set up the photo shot like this to increase sales?

Another curiosity here is the ruling about traffic offences. If there are any outstanding parking fines or speeding tickets you are not allowed to leave the country. I can see that is probably fair enough, except that no one tells you that you have committed an offence. Therefore before travelling it is essential to visit the Traffic Violation Website, log in your car registration and see if you have offended. Lionel did this for me last week as a joke and was highly amused to find that I had been done for speeding. Needless to say, I swiftly paid the fine, which was administratively a doddle. Worked first time!

Now that we're 'official' with our Residence Permits, driving licences and bank accounts, our farmhouse in the English countryside seems a long way away.

4

SANCTUARY IN THE DESERT

A t last, after three months, we have the house! But no furniture, no fridge, no cooker and everything is covered in a thick layer of fine dust. Our priority is to have the house deep cleaned in readiness for delivery of white goods and furniture, bought locally, a feat that brings its own challenges and surprises.

A cleaning company is recommended so I phone to arrange something. I hit a blank with all phone numbers, then amazingly someone rings back. She tells me in rapid broken English that she can send five Filipina women the next day. They will supply the tools but I must buy the cleaning materials.

She is also very insistent that I should meet her staff at a supermarket on one of the major roads. I explain that my knowledge of the geography of Doha is scant, that I have no idea where she means. However, I describe the nearest big landmarks: three schools, a driving school and a mosque. Since there are mosques everywhere this is probably unhelpful, but I also give our proximity to one of the ring roads and I provide the address. No one is ever interested in the address. I tried to explain our location on a map once and was roundly remonstrated with, "Don't talk to me about maps!" To be fair, he had a point since the maps are all out of date and half the street names have changed anyway.

All directions rest on narrative and proximity to big landmarks such as petrol stations where there are fast food chains. The sat nav usually shows a blip in the middle of nowhere and there is no postal system as we know it, simply a central repository of PO boxes.

So on the morning of our cleaning arrangement, we hold little hope of ever seeing them without some further discussion. Imagine our astonishment when at eight o'clock sharp, a car draws up and out tumble five diminutive Filipina maids dressed in identical pink tabards with the cleaning company's logo emblazoned on the front.

They twitter like a flock of pink budgies and set to work. They request a stepladder for the chandelier (personally I would have described it as a light but this is not a time for quibbling). One of the blue-overalled men from the construction company produces a stepladder and within minutes we encounter one of the girls at the top of the ladder, leaning out of an upstairs window so that she can clean the outside. The health and safety implications of this manoeuvre are too horrible to contemplate, so we leave them to it and go off to the furniture souq with our friends from Manchester.

Lionel has to visit the utilities office personally in order to arrange for the house to be connected to water and electricity and Mr Khalid in Housing gives him instructions on how to locate it. He's told to start at the Ramada roundabout, which is unhelpful since he doesn't know where that is, but even more unhelpful when it is explained to him that actually there is no roundabout there anymore, nor is there a Ramada hotel, which has been demolished. So he has to find a random set of traffic lights where there used to be a hotel and a roundabout. Amazingly he succeeds, although it still takes several cajoling and pleading calls before we are connected to running water.

We all have a tendency to moan about Health and Safety back at home but here it is virtually non-existent. There are vast armies of blue-overalled construction workers. They cover their heads and faces with scarves to keep off the sun and dust and can be seen in the numerous Tata buses going home to their dormitory villages, which by all accounts are extremely squalid.

Our own particular man lives in a hut on site and he is probably lucky. Whenever we arrive at the house he appears from nowhere and follows us around in case we need anything. We had a lot of trouble connecting to water and electricity and although he could do nothing about the former, a large spanner on the electricity company's box seemed to do the trick so that we had power, although he switches it off when we go.

The problem seems to be a dispute between the hospital and the landlord, but eventually the housing man at the hospital and the landlord resolve their differences and a car from the utilities company pulls up outside the house. It is driven by a Qatari, with three Qatari passengers who sit there while an Indian worker leaps out and fixes our water connection and I proffer grateful thanks to them all. Of course the next day, although our huge water tank in the courtyard is full, we still have no water flowing out of the taps.

A blue-overalled man, head moving in a vigorous figure of eight, calls his boss and suddenly there are blue-overalled men everywhere: one on the roof, one walking along a narrow twelve-foot high wall from next door, another inside. The wall-walker is leaping from the wall onto the top of the water tank whereupon he produces some tools and starts dismantling the wiring in order to get the pump to work.

This makes me very nervous, with visions of electrocution and worries about my resuscitation skills. But at least I'm assured that the electricity has been switched off and sure enough in a few minutes we have a filling header tank and functioning hot and cold running water, electricity and air conditioning. Oh joy!

This miracle hadn't happened at the time of the deep clean and our visit to the souq had been interrupted by the cleaning company boss phoning me in a state of agitation because the water had run out. We'd hastily finished our business in the souq and returned to the villa where we found that the cleaners had drained the water from the header tank but were calmly brushing the courtyard and the inside was spotless.

Everyone was happy. They smiled and chattered and asked me if I was a Christian like them. They were delighted by my affirmative reply although I failed to mention the lapsed Catholicism, which was probably an unnecessary detail. In Doha itself there are only mosques: all the places of worship for other faiths – Catholic, Orthodox, Protestant, and Jewish – are out of town, near the industrial zone.

I paid the cleaners the equivalent of about £200 for twenty-six hours work in total, Lionel slipped them a tip and they gathered on the pavement to await their car.

The house is clean but not yet liveable. We still need furniture and communication. We are expected to organise all this ourselves and the rule of three certainly applies.

Signing up for a telephone is a case in point. The

service includes television and internet access and we are helped by a charming Qatari lady who guides us through the process of filling in the form. Then she stuns us by asking for our nearest landline. We tell her that there will be plenty and name the nearby school and mosque so that she can look it up. She looks at us in amazement and informs us that she has no access to those numbers and we must find a neighbour with a telephone then return to her office with the number so that she can process the order for connection.

We wonder if this is an elaborate hoax until we hear a customer at the next booth being given the same instruction.

Still, it makes us go and knock at a neighbour's door, which is a good introduction and they fully understand about the phone number. We return to the telephone company's office where the nice Arab lady tells us, "Now you will await a phone call giving you a date for installation." So far, so good, except that we receive no call.

So Lionel phones and is informed that our account has been cancelled. Furious, I march over to see our helpful lady who investigates and apologises that the back office have failed to do their bit.

"But I will do it now and all will be well," she says.

Several phone calls and two further trips to the office and we now have a date fixed.

Handsets are not part of the package so we buy a couple in the supermarket only to discover that they are not compatible with the wall sockets. This is a triumph for British marketing as all the phones sold here have European connections but all the wall sockets are British Telecom standard. Another trip to find telephone adaptors is necessary. Lionel volunteers and finds a helpful specialist telephone/electrical store where they attempt to change the connection on the phone.

The wrong plug is cut off, leaving bare wires, and a new correct one attached … which doesn't work. So the process is repeated – several times. By now the cable from the telephone is considerably shorter than when they started but eventually it works. They beam up at him.

"We can do all your house wiring for you sir! No problem!"

We decline that offer. Meanwhile we are still waiting for our landline and internet connection.

What is the house like? It is brand new and part of a block of eighteen identical *villas*, as they call them, next to the mosque and school, with a building site opposite. We were originally offered what we'd describe as a town house, in a compound, with other European ex-pats. Status is everything round here and although we were entitled to a much larger villa, with its own swimming pool, none were available. (A swimming pool is less desirable than you might think as the water gets so hot). The town house compound option was OK, but we had been tipped off to ask if there were any stand-alone ones.

"Certainly," said Khalid, the housing manager, "but they are in the Arab style. Are you still interested?"

"But of course," we reply, intrigued by what he means.

The house is semi-detached, with servants' quarters outside as a separate building at the back. We've a double car-port at the front with electric doors operated by a zapper from the car. There's a pedestrian front gate with an answerphone to the house and the whole property is surrounded by a high wall. The 'garden' is completely tiled apart from a narrow eighteen-inch border of dirt, hardly soil, inside the front wall. I can already envisage frothy fountains of fuchsia-pink bougainvillea tumbling over this wall, but perhaps my imagination is too vivid.

Currently I doubt even bindweed would grow there. The house is double fronted, with wide marble steps leading up to a square porch. White pillars grace the corners and we've a well-appointed wooden front door with adjoining brass latticework. The walls inside and out are painted cream and white and there is a terracotta pantiled roof, although there is a flat element to the roof also, which is accessed from the back via a fire escape ladder fixed to the wall. The numerous satellite dishes are tastefully hidden from view.

Inside, the house is spacious, an open plan with a large wooden archway between the reception room, from which the front door opens, and the dining room. This latter room is almost thirty-seven metres square and has the staircase coming off from one side and large sliding French windows that open onto a shaded raised outside dining area. The somewhat unusual feature of this room is the washbasin in the corner, presumably something to do with pre-prandial ablutions. The other concession to what we presume is 'Arab style' is that all the bathrooms and lavatories have hosepipes and drains in the floor.

We have noticed this in the hospital; constantly wet floors in the loos and hosepipes by every lavatory bowl. There is a reasonable kitchen and utility room, a separate room that would do for a TV room, with its own bathroom and hosepipe (just in case) and upstairs, four large bedrooms each with an en-suite, a huge landing big enough for a couple of sofas, and a balcony.

We are expected to have live-in help. For about two thousand riyals per month (about £400), they would live in the servants' quarters: the air-conditioned room is a reasonable size with an en-suite bathroom. However, we do not want a live-in maid and instead we elect to convert the 'servants' quarters' into a gym.

All the floors are marble and the finish is good. The house has a feeling of space and light and we love it!

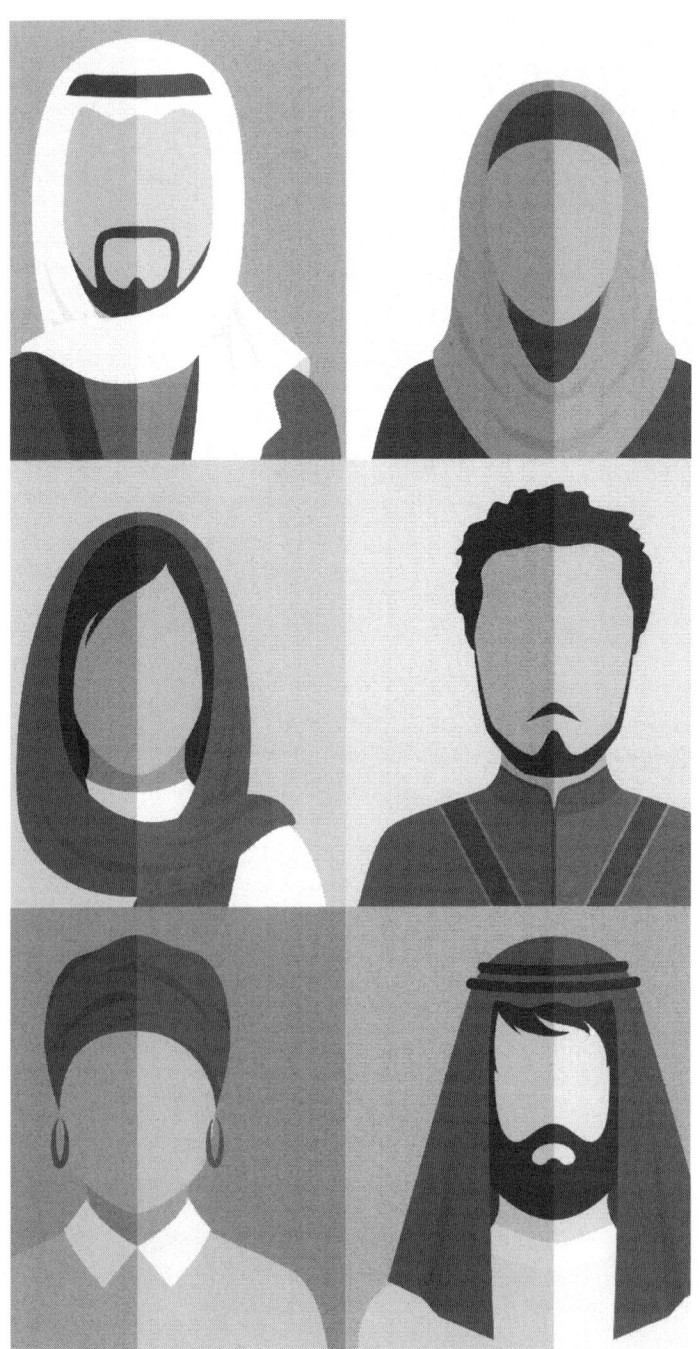

44

5

DAILY RHYTHMS

After a few months of living here, life has settled into a
rhythm. We are awoken by the first call to prayer,
which is currently at 3.30am. Our alarm goes off just
after five and we are in our cars, driving through the busy
traffic, about an hour later. From the moment the car door
closes all systems are on high alert. Dodging the numerous
accidents and taking short cuts across bits of desert scrub is
the norm. We are being constantly bombarded by blasting
horns because of a nanosecond's delay at the traffic lights.
Our arrival at work is a blessed relief.

The surprising thing is that the trip has become less
fraught with time, although no less intense. We both now
have our own designated parking places with our names
displayed above them on the sheltered canopy that shades
the steering wheel from the sun, otherwise it would be
literally too hot to handle and would need cooling with
splashes from a bottle of water kept in the car for such
purpose.

Everyone makes a point of greeting me. Ibrahim

arrives with my cup of coffee and the day begins. As a deputy chief in the corporate offices, I am essentially deputy corporate medical director for the whole corporation and every day brings different issues. I make a point of going out to the eight hospitals in the group, three of which are situated away from Doha, although I do have colleagues who summon people to their offices at corporate headquarters (and then they wonder why the staff aren't properly engaged).

At our home, domestic life has also settled into a comfortable rhythm with Agnes the maid coming four days a week, the drinking-water cooler man twice a week and the cockroach exterminator men once a month. Agnes twitters around in her pink tabard and drives me mad. She constantly forgets things, unplugs the phone and leaves the hosepipe on, but she is an excellent and conscientious cleaner. It is impossible to be angry as she giggles disarmingly and says, "Sorry, madam".

Lionel and I agree that our house is probably the most peaceful that we have ever lived in. This is partly because there are no other responsibilities such as children, pets or maintenance, but the clean lines contribute to the feeling of tranquillity. I marvel at our spacious rooms, spare elegant furniture and cool marble floors all enclosed by the high walls surrounding our courtyards. Driving back from the frenetic shopping mall, reaching home where we metaphorically pull up the drawbridge, settling down to a cool glass of sparkling wine, sitting on our veranda, gazing at a new crescent moon in the Arabian sky ... all this is peace indeed.

We're gradually becoming acclimatised to the intense heat and humidity, in fact probably more so than the Arabs who hardly go outside but live constantly cocooned in air-conditioned splendour. As a result they suffer from obesity and its concomitant diseases of diabetes and cardiovascular disease, plus vitamin D deficiency.

Even a trip to the shops, for an Arab, does not involve venturing outside. Arriving at one of the huge shopping malls, it is not unusual to see the Indian driver of a large Land Cruiser seemingly oblivious to the chaos he has caused by simply stopping outside the main entrance. The reason becomes clear when out of the back, unseen through the tinted windows, emerge several abaya-clad women of different sizes and ages. Of course they all sport designer handbags and sunglasses, and totter on spindly heels as they make their way into the cool mall by the shortest distance possible. The children follow accompanied by their Filipina nannies, who are dressed in a uniform of pyjamas with their heads covered. The 'thobelets', as we call them, are the sweetest little boys imaginable, similar to choir boys in their long robes. They parade the malls behind their big brothers, the adolescent 'thobes' who somehow have lost that charm.

Public displays of affection are frowned upon here but the rules are not straightforward so holding hands and kissing members of the same sex is absolutely fine. I am touched to see a young Arab man complete with thobe and ghuttra walking along holding hands with his heavily pregnant wife who is completely covered in black abbaya and veil. The sexes are so often completely segregated that this simple human act of affection is noticeable.

The vitamin deficiency here is certainly not dietary related. In spite of the lack of agriculture in this desert country, the supermarket shelves are well stocked. We choose simple food: fresh fruit, tasty small courgettes and cucumbers, delicious tomatoes and excellent fresh fish and meat (beef, veal, lamb and chicken). We never see any chickens so I don't know where they come from and would rather not think about it too much. The Moroccan fishmonger in the supermarket greets me like an old friend and is happy to shell half a kilo of fresh prawns for me, which I turn into a delicious dish with red chillies, garlic, fresh ginger, limes and coconut milk. Dairy produce in the guise of yoghurt and laban, a sort of yoghurt milk, is good and the eggs are unbelievable tasty.

There is an interesting local cheese, which is very salty and shaped in a coil as if made from a skein of wool. We think it might be from camel milk and due to its shape, Lionel calls it camel bollock cheese (he doesn't eat it), never mind the biological impossibility.

We are still surprised at the heat that greets us as we open the door to the outside. Leaving hotels and shops where the air-conditioning is set too high, the warm air is welcome and we love being able to eat supper outside under the stars. Weekends are a time to relax, work out in our personal gym, read and write. I play jazz on my saxophone and practise for our band sessions. To call it a band is probably stretching a point: there are five middle-aged men on guitars and drums and me on sax. Nevertheless we have a willing audience of small children who dance along to our scratch tunes while their nannies watch from the sidelines. The parents sensibly keep well away. Lionel enjoys cool showers, which is a problem since the water in the outside tank heats up and is never cold: we are considering installing a water cooler. Swimming pools in hotels have to be artificially cooled or it is like swimming in soup.

If all that sounds too impossibly boring, there are plenty of extra-curricular activities such as jazz in the big hotels, classical music concerts, restaurants, beach and other pursuits such as dune bashing which we still haven't indulged in. Young Arab men are particularly keen on this dangerous pastime. They set off in their cars across the desert, often at night, up and down the dunes like switchbacks and sadly have been known to crash into each other at the summits since there are no designated roads. Rolling over is also common as they ascend the steep-sided dunes. We are happy to give it a miss.

At work, English is the common language but many people speak Arabic and other languages abound. We have interpreters in Thai, Urdu, Tamil, Hindi, Tagalog and many more. We find the workers from the East and from the Indian sub-continent to be uncomfortably subservient and our clinical colleagues find that difficult when dealing with multi-disciplinary teams. Although meetings with Arabs can become very heated there is also a reluctance to confront people directly and it is important not to lose face. Discussions at meetings tend to drift away from the agenda, but gradually return to the topic although decisions and action points are not always easy to pin down.

Then there is appalling mobile phone etiquette. No one switches off and people answer their phones openly in meetings, then drift in and out of the room. Mobile phone numbers are happily given to patients by their doctors and no one minds being phoned in the middle of a busy clinic. Emails might be ignored but simply turning up at someone's office is perfectly acceptable. There is an element of learned helplessness that I first noticed when I arrived: people come and see us with problems then expect us to find the solution. The notion of working on something together is quite alien to many of our staff. Numerous projects start, but finishing is not a strong suit.

Political correctness is just not part of the lexicon and wouldn't be understood as a concept. Asking a woman about her children, pregnancy plans and childcare arrangements is simply expected as part of the interview process for a new job. It fascinates me that many of our British colleagues fall into local ways almost too easily, but not in a good way. I have noticed – as have several of my female colleagues – that there is an element of misogyny amongst the British males. It is almost as if they think they don't have to worry about that any more, which is very disappointing. It's also a contrast to the Arabs who do seem to respect us for the job that we are doing.

But there is life outside the hospital too. Shopping, like many activities, is done after dark. The large shopping malls, of which there are many, are open during the day but the souqs only come to life in the evenings.

Souqs at first glance appear to be chaotic places, but it swiftly becomes apparent that there *is* an order, which is a group of shops all selling similar wares. We noticed this first in Dubai years ago when we visited the gold souq, which is opulent in the extreme.

Wandering along the less salubrious old souq here, not far from the harbour with its former pearl-diving dhows, we find the fabric souqs, the antique artefacts souq (especially for the foreigners) and hidden in narrow alleyways, useful souqs like the nuts and bolts souq, hardware souq and less useful, caged birds souq. These birds are songbirds or parrots and many of them sport such exotic plumage in such vivid fluorescent colours that I wonder if their feathers are dyed.

However, best not to dwell on such things especially when a toothless old Arab turns to me proffering a large green lizard for sale. I politely decline and hurry on past. Eventually I find the fabric souq that is my destination. This is a maze of shops within a covered area, not unlike a European market. The fabrics are sumptuous silks in rich jewel-like colours, fine cottons, sari fabrics, good quality linens in plain colours, and there is so much choice it is difficult to know where to start. There is a very high bling factor, so it is difficult to find something without gold or silver trim, but with perseverance it can be done.

Bargaining is expected and even while I am browsing, the vendor will be negotiating the price. I buy some silk in emerald green with fuchsia pink spots for a jacket plus a swathe of excellent quality boucle cotton for a Chanel type suit, with a plan to have such a suit made at the tailor, having given him a suit to copy.

Having finally made my purchase I then go along to the tailor with my knowledgeable friend, Moira, cousin of a friend from home, who has been teaching out there for years and who makes the introductions. The tailor's place is in a scruffy road and he is surrounded by other tailors, many of whom seem to specialise in thobes, which is presumably a limited skill since they all look the same. But doubtless there are numerous variations, even if they are all long and white. As we cross the threshold of our tailor's front door I am enchanted to find, in true sartorial fashion, a group of tailors sitting cross-legged on the floor working on garments, some of which are being intricately embroidered.

I imagine this is a scene that has remained largely unchanged since the Middle Ages.

The expert cutters, one of whom is recommended by Moira, stand behind long tables and I produce my Paris-purchased suit and ask him if he can copy it in my newly bought fabric. He appraises the fabric and gives his approval, then frowns while we discuss details such as the skirt length (just below mid-calf for work) and the not inconsiderable details on the jacket, then he makes a few scribbled sketches on a notepad and gives me a price, whereupon I leave a deposit in cash, and we fix a date for collection.

The day of reckoning is due and Moira and I eagerly meet at the tailors. She's completely addicted to this process and has a wardrobe full of beautifully cut linen skirts and jackets. The tailor produces my suit, which is expertly tailored with all original details and it fits me perfectly. Everyone in the establishment is impressed including two Arab women who are waiting their turn in the tiny changing cubicle. We presume they are having something made to wear under their black abeyas but they give nothing away. The price is very reasonable and he gets my business for the silk jacket, which I collect the following week.

Specialist souqs – such as the chaotic furniture-making souq – are located in different areas of the city. Our friends Sohaib and Sadhia take us and they have the distinct advantage over us in that although they were both born and bred in Manchester, their parents were originally from Pakistan. We have never been there but assume that this is a microcosm of it. Sohaib and Sadhia are fluent in the appropriate languages and negotiate for wardrobes on our behalf.

The chaos begins when we arrive in the square around which all the souq's warehouses and workshops are situated. We simply stop the cars at random and alight, whereupon there is much shouting and gesticulation so we get back in, drive another twenty yards or so and stop again. This must be acceptable since no objections ensue. When we try to leave, we are blocked in but this is not a major problem since there is a huge commotion, much shouting and running in and out of buildings and a driver is found who moves the offending vehicle. We have been delayed about two minutes. The system, chaotic as it appears, does seem to work.

The workshop owner proudly tells us that his

wardrobes are made of "the finest MDF wood" skilfully painted in two colours to resemble mahogany. We order three in different sizes and all is agreed, while the two wives are made to sit on rickety three-legged stools produced for our benefit. We both mutter that writing something down might be a good idea (but to no avail) and sip our hot, milky, sweet tea. It is revolting but has to be drunk out of politeness.

Again, a price is agreed, deposits in cash are paid and a week later a battered pick-up truck draws up at the house with a pile of filthy mattresses on a trailer.

"We have your wardrobes," announces the driver proudly. I view the scene with dismay until I realise that the mattresses are protecting the panels of the wardrobes, which are carefully unloaded and taken upstairs on the heads of the workmen.

We have four possible bedrooms upstairs and they clearly think I am eccentric by wanting all the wardrobes constructed in one room. This is all part of our cunning plan to turn a six-bedroomed house into a one-bedroomed one. So five bedrooms become one dressing room, two studies (one each), a gym and a television room leaving us with one spacious minimalist bedroom. The wardrobes are neither solid nor beautiful but they are spacious and functional, make a perfect dressing room, and within forty minutes, the job is done.

Although we are enjoying decorating our spacious house with a mixture of western minimalism and the occasional Arab artefact (the effect is eclectic but seems to work), the paved courtyard enclosed by twelve-foot-high walls is less appealing. It does have marble steps up to the front door and a shady terrace at the back that will accommodate a breakfast table. There is a strip of sandy dirt below a north-east facing wall and although I still have visions of tumbling bougainvillea growing along this wall, that prospect now seems unlikely. Nevertheless we make an attempt at a garden to break up the stark walls and lack of colour.

At the garden centre, Suman – a small wiry Nepalese who speaks good English (he used to be a tourist guide in the Himalayas) – volunteers to come to the house to advise on plants.

"When?" I ask.

"Now," he says, whereupon he hops into our car and off we go.

I can't quite believe that I might grow my own lemons but of course in this climate, provided there is water, this poses no problem. With Suman we draw up plans for the judicious placing of pots and planters and the next day an army of Nepalese gardeners appear with trees, shrubs, small plants and masses of compost, which they proceed to assemble into a courtyard garden.

Six weeks later the gardeners are back to trim the topiary shrubs next to the terrace and to fertilise the plants. The bougainvillea is not yet tumbling over the wall but it has produced long tendrils supporting deep pink, purple and creamy white leaves with tiny white flowers amidst them. Technically the colour of this plant comes from the new leaves and the flowers are the least impressive feature. We also have lollipop trees, which have a canopy of different shades of bougainvillea, all of which have been grafted onto a thick trunk.

These specimens, which are quite splendid, are imported from Valencia in Spain, as is the olive tree which we have sited in front of a garden wall light so in the evening the light is filtered through its green canopy. The effect is stunning and with the heady scent from the lemon blossom, the arid, stark courtyard is now transformed into a magical haven beyond the desert scrubland outside.

We are determined not to suffer from vitamin D deficiency, so we gently top up our tans for a couple of hours each weekend, and keep the osteomalacia (a softening of the bones caused by lack of vitamin D) at bay. The sunloungers and sun umbrella blend in with our plants and although there is no pool, we are content in our private space. Pools are difficult to maintain for much of the year, since they need to be artificially cooled or they reach the temperature of a hot bath – hardly refreshing.

Around the city are municipal gardens, beautifully maintained with long avenues of palm trees, frangipani and tropical hedges. Splashes of colour from petunias line the road and at the entrance to the hospital, where gardeners are a continual presence, although weeding is not an onerous task since few weeds grow in the unrelenting heat. As I drive into work in the morning, one particular gardener, who sports an exuberant turban and is dressed in baggy khaki trousers tucked into his wellingtons, always greets me with a cheery grin and wave.

Occasionally he thrusts a bunch of newly picked mint leaves into my hands with the instruction, "Make chai. Very good chai."

Once, while sitting in the traffic, I observed tree-planting in progress. There were two men down a hole, a supervisor, two apparent under-supervisors, tree-handling people and several observers. In total I counted twelve men to plant one tree. This was not a large tree but a mere sapling and I reflected that it was the sort of tree that the average British Dad would pick up from the garden centre one Saturday afternoon, load onto the roof-rack, head home, dig a hole and have it planted in time for a self-satisfied beer before supper.

Similarly when the exact position of our olive tree was

not quite right, it took three of them to move it, plus one giving orders. After they had left it still wasn't correct, so Lionel just shifted it on his own with no trouble. It is not a case of strength; when our cooker was delivered – a large electric oven and hob all in one – the tiny Nepalese delivery man, who could have been no more than five feet tall, carried it in on his back, effortlessly, up the front door steps and into our kitchen.

Labour is cheap and there are always several people to do a job that at home we would tend to do ourselves. There is also a pecking order, so when Suman, the boss, was assessing one of our plants, he indicated one of his underlings should plunge his hand into the soil whereupon they both looked at the scooped up handful of dirt, scrutinised it, sniffed it, almost tasted it, before declaring it fine. The boss's hands remained scrupulously clean.

The introduction of flora into the garden has brought an unexpected bonus of fauna. There are very few insects around, presumably because it is so hot and dry, but we see bee-like creatures feasting on our lemon blossom and doubtless facilitating cross-pollination with a neighbour's tree. Yesterday there was a distressed damsel fly, or similar, flying round the kitchen but we managed to free it and watched as it made its way to the spindly plants surrounding our water butt.

To our amazement, we then realised that there were several of these creatures resting on the plants, cleverly disguised to look like twigs. Our zoological knowledge lets us down but it appears that we have created a haven for stick insects.

6

PIDGIN ENGLISH

There are advantages to living near the Al Khebra driving school, the main one being that most delivery men seem to know it and therefore can, in theory, find our house. The disadvantages become apparent when they fail to follow the simple instructions from the driving school to our house and Lionel is asked to go and meet them at the school (it really isn't far or difficult; we can see it from our upstairs windows).

Finding a white van outside a Middle Eastern driving school at changeover time is probably one of the most dangerous tasks on the planet. Given that the learner drivers are being deposited by their families at break-neck speed, it is also a difficult task, while the learners finishing their lessons are gingerly driving back and being collected by different families, who park in the usual random fashion. Most of them also seem to drive white vans.

Driving around the neighbourhood is also fraught with danger as the driving school offers tuition for bus drivers and lorry drivers. Accidents happen. We were waiting for our curtain makers to arrive, with me standing in the road, mobile phone glued to my ear as I tried to guide them in, unsuccessfully, when one of our neighbours came to help. Abandoning his family by their car, he took my phone and proceeded to give the same instructions in Urdu, while disappearing off along the road to the mosque with Lionel, as it appeared that was where the curtain makers were headed.

Lionel and neighbour arrived at the mosque to find complete chaos. One of the worshippers had been run over by a learner driver, there were sirens blaring along with the muezzin's call to prayer and no sign of the curtain makers. Our neighbour was still berating them on my phone when they sheepishly emerged from the mosque, where they had stopped, not to pray, but to have a pee. Thankfully the worshipper was not badly hurt.

The other good landmark for finding us is the local petrol station. Everyone seems to know it, probably because of its array of tacky fast-food shops. Directions from it are very straightforward assuming you are driving past it on the main road. Unfortunately it is impossible to exit the petrol station directly onto the main road. Instead there are a myriad of routes through the fast-food shops, with one-way signs which are completely ignored so that eventually you find your way out of a back entrance and if you go the wrong way, end up looking at the main road from the blind end of a cul-de-sac.

I was judiciously making a three-point-turn at this point when a tiny car zoomed past me and proceeded to venture off-road through the desert whereupon I saw him literally tumble onto the main road causing several vehicles to swerve and screech their brakes. Suffice it to say, the best way to direct people from Abu Hamour petrol station is to go and find them among the fast-food outlet melee.

Our recent foray into the legal field over here also gave us a link to the driving school. For various complicated reasons involving having a part delivered to our boat in Turkey, we had to have a document attested by a Notary Public – and quickly, as the Turkish customs would not release the goods. We were advised that the embassy could do this, but not on Boxing Day and although we know the Ambassador, we thought that contacting him to sort out our yacht was pushing our luck! Luckily we discovered a local lawyer who proudly advertised his location near the Al Khebra driving school.

The Turks were happy with an Arabic lawyer, so Lionel made an appointment and pitched up. The lawyer proudly told him about the business he had in relation to the driving school, either pupils complaining about their instructors or victims of accidents complaining about the pupils. It all had a ring of truth. The lawyer duly witnessed, signed and stamped our document, whereupon Lionel noticed that he was also a magician.

As his clerk was summoned after Lionel had paid the fee, the hundred riyal note was deftly thrust into the long pocket of his thobe and the rest of the documentation handed over. No one pays any tax, so who knows what dodgy business he was doing, but from our point of view it worked. The subsequent story in Turkey was less satisfactory with a multitude of sharp practices by customs, courier company and lorry drivers before we finally received our goods.

In the eternal traffic jams, we listen to the radio. There is an English speaking-station that is broadcast by the national broadcasting company. It is certainly not the BBC World Service nor Radio Four but it has news bulletins, music and chanting. The latter is the call to prayer, which interrupts whatever is being broadcast at the time. The music is generally dreadful and the disc jockeys unbelievably anodyne. Lionel has a view that they are the rejects from Radio 1, but he is being kind.

The news is certainly different. Bulletins are brief, preceded by a spot of martial music before the 7am newsreader comes on air. She has a beautiful mellow voice with perfect English pronunciation but seems to read the Arabic names with an authentic accent too. There is little time for much news after the escapades of the Emir, Sheikha and other sundry members of the Royal family have been reported. These might be as exciting as congratulating the new president of the USA on his re-election and every announcement is made very formally, so for example:

"His Highness, Sheikh Hamad bin Khalifa Al Thani sent letters of congratulation to President Obama on the occasion of his re-election as president. The Prime Minister, His Excellency, Sheikh ... bin ... Al Thani also sent letters of congratulation."

Names are very long, with the given name first, followed by the father's, followed by the family name. There are a few notable powerful families and the main offices of state tend to be taken by members of the same (Royal) family. *Bin* means son of and *Bint*, daughter of. Given names often have a theme; for example I attended a meeting last week with an Abdul theme. There was an Abdul, an Abdulla, an Abdulaziz, an Abdulattif and an Abdulmajid, so once you get the hang of it, it becomes quite easy.

We have taken to early rising since moving into our house. This allows us to miss the traffic in the morning but also means that we miss the music and get the Middle Eastern equivalent of Thought or Prayer for the Day – for an hour. It starts with thirty minutes of reading from the

Holy Qur'an, delivered in perfect BBC English. Actually it is quite interesting and philosophically there is a lot of sense, a few parables and a few references to Old Testament figures such as Moses, Noah and Abraham.

The next broadcast comprises readings from the life of the Prophet (may peace be upon him). The brackets are because this phrase is used after every reference to Mohammed the Prophet (may be peace be upon him), which makes for a somewhat turgid narrative. Yesterday there was a long piece about whether it was forbidden to eat lizards or not. The answer was that it was allowed but the Prophet himself (may peace be upon him) didn't really like them so declined the lizard meat when offered. This straightforward message took about fifteen minutes on air as we heard about Miriam, daughter of etc. etc. who had cooked a lizard, then someone else who wondered about the probity of eating lizards, all the while punctuated by the appropriate offering of peace.

It is a good illustration of how religion is closely woven into the fabric of daily life. Apart from missing the traffic, the real reason for getting up early is the dawn call to prayer. Our local man from the mosque at the end of the road is very loud, very enthusiastic and very persistent. Just when you think it is all over and are trying to snooze with head stuffed firmly under pillow, he starts up again and there is no escape. Easier simply to get up and get going, with a spot of religion to help you on your way. The broadcast is punctuated with bursts of beautiful Arabian music.

I was listening to this as I drove along a dusty road with the sun just rising, giving everything a dusky rose-coloured hue. An old man in a long white robe wearing a turban tied in the Omani style was wandering along the desert scrub closely followed by a girl dressed in a shalwar kameez (long shirt and baggy trousers) of vibrant oranges and reds. These different nationalities and styles of dress have now become commonplace to us, but observing it while listening to such haunting music exemplified what a different world this is to our green, gently undulating Hampshire valley.

I am not given to homesickness but am occasionally knocked sideways by small things such as sea-shanties being played on the radio. Suddenly I find myself missing dank, cold misty mornings, winter evenings around the fire and muddy walks over the fields and stiles. Temporary homesickness. When we did go home on leave, we soon missed the warmth of the desert.

We never missed the traffic or the driving. The school run is definitely something to be avoided, particularly at home time. Our local English town of Bishops Waltham is fairly chaotic with parents parking along the road and the lollipop lady stopping the traffic at frequent intervals, but at least the cars are parked in an orderly fashion with deference given to those with right of way. In Qatar there is no concept of a right of way and pedestrians take to the roads unwillingly (unless they are certifiably mad).

So when school is out, the cars are randomly parked on the adjacent scrubland. Parents march their children through the cars, which move in any direction like Brownian motion – completely random. I witness this in horror and watch aghast as the school gates open and about fifteen school buses, conveying about thirty children apiece, drive out in parallel formation. I say parallel but this configuration does not last long before the buses start vying for a place on the road, criss-crossing each other, blasting their horns while a few policemen try vainly to stop the utter carnage which I am convinced is about to ensue.

Each bus could be considered a competitor at the start of a cross-country run: a long journey ahead, and essential to win psychological advantage by pushing the competition off the track – any injury would simply be an unintended consequence. We are surrounded by schools and it is the same at all of them. Somehow everyone survives.

The builders are everywhere. We live opposite a building site where we are privileged every Saturday morning to hear the pile-driver digging the foundations for the new houses opposite ours, thereby precluding a gentle lie-in. The rate at which the buildings progress is remarkable. This is partly due to the numerous workers who toil day and night. At one stage I count thirty workmen on the roof of a moderate sized house opposite ours.

Driving home today in the dark, I was sitting in the traffic and struck by the work proceeding by spotlight on the new monorail system. The traffic was composed of new Land Cruisers and fast sports cars, all driven by Arabs in full thobe and ghutra. A few westerners like me drive similar cars; these are interspersed with buses taking labourers home to their camps. Unlike our cars which are all air-conditioned, the buses have open windows, and have often seen life elsewhere, such as the old yellow school buses from America which still have legends on their doors exhorting motorists to watch out for children.

The labourers, as they are unashamedly called, are frequently fast asleep, with heads lolling onto shoulders. They look exhausted, which is unsurprising considering the hard physical work they do in conditions of intense heat.

There is a shortage of housing for the ever-increasing population here that partly explains the building boom, but the other major factor is the soccer World Cup which is being hosted here in 2022.

Locals are given land when they marry and have

children, so they build new houses. Some of these are extremely extravagant such as the palace that is being built next to a roundabout on my route home. You might imagine that this is not the ideal spot for a grand house: not only is there a large roundabout but also a complicated double flyover feeding traffic onto the cross-city highway.

Location, location, location is the mantra of estate agents, yet this couldn't be a worse spot - unless you want easy access to the motorway perhaps? In truth, we believe that the locals don't care. Not remotely interested in the outdoors, their gardens are small and all grandeur is carefully secreted inside in heavily air-conditioned surroundings.

With this in mind we were amused by a recent review of Psychiatry services where recommendations from the UK Royal College were invoked, one of which was that psychiatric in-patients would benefit from some gentle gardening. The Psychiatric building is located in the middle of two dual carriageways, surrounded by a bit of desert and the thought that patients might wish to grow a few radishes or tend the roses in such an environment is truly laughable.

The palace is still in concrete form but the elements of diverse architectural styles can be clearly seen. There are grand porticos, columns, arches, domes and a few random turrets for good measure. Some palaces employ more recognisable styles such as the exact replica of the military staff college at Sandhurst that is situated on the main road next to one of the more extravagant shopping malls. This particular mall has fake Venetian buildings, clouds painted on the ceilings and indoor canals with battery-powered gondolas driven by Filipinos in stripy shirts.

From the road, as I watch the labourers attacking the ground with pickaxes, while listening to Mozart on my car stereo, I wonder about the difference in our lives. The labourers undoubtedly earn more than in their home countries but nevertheless, they are indentured workers, virtually slaves. A recent newspaper article stated:

The International Trade Union Confederation slammed the country as a "21st-century slave state" earlier this year over its alleged poor conditions for guest workers and human rights abuses. The world's leading union claimed that 191 Nepali workers died in Qatar in 2010, most of them because of heart attacks caused by outdoor temperatures rising to up to 50C.

We know that living conditions for such workers are poor and when they do arrive in hospital, there are often angry scenes if they are seen by a doctor before a local patient, even when triage shows their needs are more urgent. This is such a pressing problem that government policy is to build several new hospitals designated *Labourers Hospitals*.

My first reaction is that this is a form of apartheid and a highly distasteful concept. Nevertheless, it would mean that these workers have equal access to healthcare and on balance it is a reasonable, pragmatic solution. Don't imagine that local doctors approve of the potential imbalance in healthcare provision: the chair of rehabilitation medicine is a feisty Qatari woman who trained in Scandinavia and works tirelessly to ensure her patients have good access to care, especially when they are discharged from hospital.

The problem is that many of the labourers are here alone, with families thousands of miles away and their accommodation is entirely unsuitable for someone with a disability. Family members are unable to visit as they cannot afford the flights, so there are repatriation schemes and charitable schemes that help such patients.

All workers here (including us) have to be sponsored, but if a worker becomes ill or injured, even as a result of an industrial accident, the companies sometimes try to absolve themselves of all responsibility.

My feisty rehab doctor has ways of dealing with this. As a senior figure in local society, with plenty of *wasta*, she simply tips off the Ministry of Labour when companies are being difficult. Somehow, her patients suddenly get a better deal.

In a society where the common language is not the mother tongue of most people, well over fifty percent of communication is non-verbal. English may be the universal language but although many seem to speak it, it soon becomes apparent that their competency is limited. To make things more difficult, the mobile phone is the main means of communication. Lionel is alarmed as he observes me offering my phone number to some random shopkeeper who hasn't even asked for it (I have to admit that said shopkeeper is a smooth, good-looking Italian!).

"Well, most people want it," I respond to his perplexed look.

Since non-verbal clues are irrelevant over the phone, conversations with non-English speakers can be difficult. Our curtain maker is a case in point. As usual he failed to turn up for an appointment on time, so I phone and get the response, "Sorry I am now remembering," which roughly translates as "Oops, I forgot".

We find ourselves speaking in Pidgin English. For example, when giving directions, we say "Go straight, go right, go left, go straight", rather than elaborating about pertinent landmarks such as traffic lights, roundabouts or similar. I have always been intrigued by the novelist Amitav Ghosh's depiction of language (in his book *Sea of Poppies*) amongst seafarers in colonial India and the Far

East; now it makes sense:

Zachary soon found himself speaking to the serang with an unaccustomed ease: it was as if his oddly patterned speech had unloosed his own tongue.
"Serang Ali, where you from?"he asked.
"Serang Ali blongi Rohingya - from Arakan-side."
"And where'd you learn that kinda talk?"
"Afeem ship,"came the answer. "Chinaside."

I am constantly astonished by the ability of other nationalities to speak English. Nonetheless, some of the expressions bring out a puerile sense of humour in me. For example, when trying to guide a recovery vehicle to my broken-down car (it had a puncture), the man on the end of the mobile phone assured me he knew where I was with the wonderful phrase, "I am looking up your backside, madam."

All in all, people generally are very courteous. We recently bought a silk Kashmiri carpet to hang on the wall. This process takes time and there is a ritual that must be followed. We are asked to sit, given jasmine tea to drink and the carpets are displayed with a great flourish. We are expected to ponder, look at certain ones again and have them turned upside down as the colours change depending on the pile. A magnifying glass and dividers are brought out so that we can accurately determine the number of knots per square inch and the longer we take on our deliberations, the more the price is reduced.

Having finally made our choice, the carpet is delivered and hung on the wall although Lionel ends up doing some DIY, since the carpet vendor, in spite of his protestations, doesn't know one end of a drill from the other. When we return to the same shop we admire the vendor's fabulously ornate copy of the Qur'an, clearly a prized possession, and from which he was reading as we arrived. Our admiration is countered by his offering the book as a gift – we decline but with difficulty.

Lionel recently drove himself up to the hospital in the north of the country. Maps are incomplete and the Sat-Nav is almost worse than useless but he had plenty of advice before he left which went along the lines of, "It's easy to find and you can't miss it".

All of this is true but only when you know where you are going. Needless to say, he was lost and stopped in the middle of the desert to consult his useless map, whereupon out of nowhere an itinerant Arab appeared wearing a grubby green thobe and carrying a roughly hewn staff. Communication was limited but the Arab pointed at the map.

"Al Khor?" he asked.

"Yes!" replied Lionel, delighted.

Within seconds the Arab had leaped into the car and sat in the passenger seat with his staff propped up between his knees. A lift wasn't exactly what Lionel had proposed but it seemed fair enough so he took him to the town, whereupon the Arab gestured where he needed dropping off, leaving Lionel still completely clueless as to the whereabouts of the hospital.

Eventually he found it and in true Arab fashion the appointments had all gone wrong but the Chief Executive was summoned from home and all was well. He even commiserated with Lionel about the difficulties of finding the place and reassured him that next time would be easier. There was no suggestion that maps or directions might be offered to newcomers in the future.

7

GOING NATIVE

It is Christmas Eve and we have already clocked up a hundred days in the Middle East, so it's a good time for reflection. It is fascinating, infuriating, at times weird, but always interesting and intriguing. The biggest revelation for me has been the character of the Arabs. If I am honest, I had never really thought much about Arabs as a race. I knew that Arabs had been slave traders so that might have coloured my thoughts and of course they are now very wealthy from oil, and there is the added fundamentalist religious aspect plus the zealous Sharia law, evident in places like Saudi Arabia.

Re-reading the last sentence, it might be construed that I harboured some sort of unspoken prejudice. Maybe I did, deep down, and if so, how very wrong I was. This Christmas season in particular has made me appreciate their warmth, generosity and hospitality. Most Europeans escape home for the festive season but we elected to stay and work as usual. This gesture was really appreciated by the locals, who gave us gifts, told us not to work at all on

Christmas Day (but we did) and one of the highly respected Arab leaders who, it is rumoured, is anti-British, loitered outside my office door, smiled at me and admonished, "You are doing all the work. All the other Britons have gone home."

Tentatively, I invited him in to sit and chat, which he did for an hour. Apparently this was a tremendous honour, hitherto almost unheard of.

However, nothing is simple, so although the Arabs are really charming, amusing and helpful to me, they are unashamedly racially prejudiced. An example is in the instructions for recruiting new members of staff: try to appoint a Qatari, failing that a Gulf Arab, failing that any other Arab, failing that, a foreigner will do. Foreigners encompass any non-Arab. However, there is a pecking order, but exactly where Filipinos come in relation to Indians and in relation to Westerners, is difficult to ascertain. I assumed that a female Brit would be pretty low down the pecking order but I am assured that this is not the case. Certainly I am treated with the utmost respect.

Interestingly, the racial prejudice is not overtly colour prejudice. Gulf Arabs can be traced from three genetic roots, Arabia, Africa and Persia. The phenotypes or observable characteristics of these peoples are very different. Those from northern Iran are often fair with blue eyes whereas those from Africa have dark skin and this diversity is evident in the Arabs. There are some who are very dark and some who with their small neat moustaches could be British bank managers from Tunbridge Wells, though with the thobe and ghutra removed obviously.

[Lionel is having difficulty coping with the prospect of a naked moustachioed Tunbridge Wells bank manager.]

Families are large, with consanguinity an issue and marriage between first cousins not uncommon. They are unashamedly tribal as explained by a consultant colleague whose elderly mother was ill and needed treatment abroad. The decision to travel was debated not by the mother or her children but by the whole extended family before eventually, they turned to my colleague saying, "You're a doctor so you can decide."

He was then able to discuss the pros and cons with his mother, who agreed to travel for the treatment. Its success meant that she was able to enjoy six more years of good quality life, go on pilgrimage and enjoy her grandchildren. A happy ending, but not without some effort on his part.

Family bonds are stronger in the Middle East than in western societies where elderly people are sometimes marginalised and end up living alone, far from their families. In spite of the flaws in Arab society I feel we can learn from them, particularly in the strength of their family ties which are genuine and not seen as an onerous duty.

Arab social mores, culture and customs are difficult to understand. I am working late when one of the office boys literally thrusts a young Arab into my office and hastily retreats. The young man, who is about thirty years old, is polite but very angry. He introduces himself, shakes my hand and voices his concerns. Apparently his wife, currently in hospital, has been examined by a male doctor. He explains that in his culture this is completely unacceptable and moreover it was an intimate examination, which makes it even worse. He feels personally violated.

We have a long discussion and he concedes that in a dire emergency, treatment of a female patient by a male doctor would be allowed. However, this is not such a case and although I hesitantly ask him if he wishes to make an official complaint, he is adamant that he does not, nor does he want to meet the doctor concerned; the implication being that if he does, he would have to kill him.

The conversation continues and the young husband appears somewhat appeased, but requests that I speak to his wife. So we go up to the Gynaecology wards, where his wife is not on her bed but we find her, a lone figure dressed in black, with her face completely covered, pacing the corridor. She is upset and I suggest going back to her room for some privacy, whereupon she leaps up onto her bed, whips off the abaya and veil and underneath is barely clad in skinny jeans and strappy T-shirt. She looks like any young woman bouncing along Oxford Street on a summer afternoon.

We discuss her concerns which are mainly around an impending MRI scan and I am able to reassure her. A vigorous discussion ensues between husband and wife about the morning's examination. It all sounds fine to me. She had been properly chaperoned, her dignity was respected, she was covered and the doctor explained everything, so in essence she had no complaints. Eventually the atmosphere eases and all seems well. The husband is appeased and both are very grateful to me for taking the time to listen and explain.

It seems appropriate to leave them so I stand up and proffer my hand to the husband, slightly hesitantly, checking, "You will shake my hand?"

"Oh yes," replies his wife. "He's very progressive."

There are two postscripts to this story. The first concerns the consultant in charge of Gynaecology radiology. She is blazing when I relate the tale and insists that I send the young man to her so that she can explain to him. She will eat him alive, even though she also is completely veiled apart from her eyes, seen through a thin slit.

The other colleague, with whom I discuss the case, is a gentle Qatari doctor in charge of patient complaints. He agrees with my approach and also explains that the husband might never have spoken to him because he is a man and the husband's honour was at stake, whereas I am no threat, being female and a westerner. Nothing is simple or predictable.

Anthropologists talk about 'going native' and I confess that in spite of my reservations about the driving here, I have done exactly that. Yesterday I found myself heading off-road onto the desert scrub in order to bypass a long queue of traffic – they all do it – undertaking a bus (a thing I would never do in the UK) and texting a colleague while sitting in traffic, as I moved slowly up to a roundabout. I have also discovered the horn.

The unusual has started to become normal, so I happily stand while someone unpacks my trolley at the supermarket checkout, puts the purchases into bags then wheels the trolley back to my car and packs the boot for me. How on earth will I cope in Tesco's when I return home?

The culmination of the first hundred days is a conference organised by me and co-hosted with a local colleague. The British have all gone home for Christmas, so Lionel and I are the only Westerners in the room. It is a tremendous success. I put them into groups, with a facilitator chosen from the group, a question posed for discussion, and a requirement for feedback. They go to the task with gusto and although the culture is different, the issues facing the medical profession are similar to those at home and the attitudes of the doctors towards their patients are the same.

I hear tales here of poor communication and lack of patient involvement, notably from the Arabs who are vociferous and demanding about their treatment, while the ex-pats – particularly the unskilled labourers – are compliant. Yet in my session the overriding concern is to improve care for our patients. Change is a fact of life out here.

His Highness the Emir and his wife Her Highness the Sheikha want to establish a 'knowledge economy' in this country and there are numerous partnerships with prestigious western universities, in stunning buildings grouped in Education City. The whole city is growing by the day, with new buildings and roads, yet only two generations ago, many of the locals were still living in the desert, possibly nomadic or scraping a living as fishermen, the pearl trade having died earlier in the twentieth century. So it is not surprising that there are conflicts, as the outer show clashes with the deep-seated traditions of this proud and ancient culture.

8

BEYOND THE VEIL

After a year of living here I sometimes get a glimpse of understanding about why the women dress as they do.

I have been told that wearing the veil gives women an anonymity that they enjoy. Personally I am not convinced and yet perhaps they enjoy the air of mystery?

The really difficult one is the niqab, which is the covering of the face so that only the eyes show. To western eyes this seems an imposition, imprisonment, and paradoxically the wearers of this garb look somewhat sinister. However, having lived and worked among such women, my views are now less clear.

Lionel has numerous members of staff who dress in this way and they are affronted if he does not recognise them. Moreover they use their eyes very expressively and often flirtatiously. We ex-pats hold up Britain as a beacon of religious and racial tolerance so were shocked at reports of a journalist wearing the niqab being verbally abused and threatened on the streets of Britain recently. Ostensibly the niqab is worn for religious reasons but I am not convinced by the portrayal of this custom in the British press. It is undoubtedly cultural and many women who wear it here dress completely differently when abroad.

The hijab, which covers the head, is different. This is worn by most Muslim women, certainly those from the Middle East and the Philippines. The covering of the head denotes religious observance, whereas the face covering would seem to represent more of a cultural phenomenon. Muslims from the Indian sub-continent tend to have a more relaxed attitude but that might just be my impression.

Iraqis, Egyptians and other non-Gulf Arab nations are as incredulous as we British are of this face-covering concept. Looking back at our own culture, covering the head was very common. In the mid-twentieth century hats were commonly worn and always in church and in Victorian times, women would usually cover their head. Maybe we contemporary women are the unusual ones in the history of civilisation.

I work with many highly educated women who wear the niqab. They have all been educated in the west and I found myself in a fascinating conversation with such a woman recently. She is a leading paediatrician, much lauded in the national press for her work with diabetic children and much photographed, except in her niqab she looks exactly like everyone else. Having lunch with her recently I remarked on her wonderful shoes, which were glitzy animal print with eye-popping platform soles and heels.

She smiled, with her eyes of course, and asked my opinion of her blouse, naming a well-known Italian designer. I had to look twice because she was wearing a long black abaya, but sure enough, peeping below the sleeves were cuffs of matching silk animal print. We then embarked on a long conversation about fashion and her love of New York where she would pass several good shops on her way to and from work. This woman is not subjugated but she chooses to dress in this way in her own country.

Another example of dress customs occurred in a local restaurant, much frequented by locals and ex-pats. It is situated within a hotel so alcohol is served. A local couple arrived and sat at a table next to me where I was eating with a female friend. The man was in traditional robes and the woman's face was completely covered by the thin gauzy niqab, which only allows vision outwards. Once settled at the table she threw her veil back to reveal a beautiful face, exquisitely made-up, and the pair carried on with their meal like any other couple out on a date. Interestingly, her back was to the restaurant so very few people would have seen her face.

Beautiful eyes do not always mean a beautiful face and I know that the promise of a beautiful face, having seen the eyes, can be a disappointment when the face fails to meet expectations. But not always.

One of Lionel's female, fully veiled, niqab-wearing members of staff came to see him about a car parking problem. It is amazing how such banal issues can inflame passions. Her interests became more obvious when she showed him a photo on her mobile phone. It was of her, wearing scanty western dress and apparently looking very beautiful. He had the sense to steer the conversation back to parking.

Women are very aware of their clothes and bodies. One of my staff was in hospital after the summer break. Naturally I was concerned but all was revealed, literally, when she bounced into my office on her return to work, and proudly opened her abaya to reveal a massive new cleavage. The dermatologists, male and female, happily

Botox each other and liposuction is a common operation.

I am given a beautiful abaya by a local friend. It is black but embroidered extravagantly with silver thread and comes with a matching shayla – a long rectangular scarf. I cannot wear the shayla without it slipping off my hair, but if I wear it loosely round my head with a bit of hair showing it looks fine and is perfectly acceptable because I am neither Muslim nor Arab.

I wore it to work, mainly to demonstrate my gratitude to my friend but I was concerned that it might be construed as disrespectful. In fact, it was the opposite. They all loved it and several photos were taken, then posted around to other colleagues. I ensured that I did the full works i.e. plenty of eye makeup, extravagant mascara, killer heels, designer sunglasses and bag. Surprisingly enough it was all quite comfortable and easy to wear, although I couldn't quite master the Arab ladies' glide. They walk very slowly, sashaying along the corridors without obviously touching the ground.

I am afraid that I hitched up my skirts and rattled along at fast pace, tripping over my heels and looking extremely inelegant as my shayla fell off and my abaya flew open.

I have been organising several workshops in a five-star hotel. Having lunch with some Arab colleagues, we are treated to a model wandering through the dining area, wearing an exquisitely embroidered dress in flaming colours. My friend Mustafa chatted to her.

"That's a beautiful dress. Is something special going on?" he asks.

"It's the Arabian fashion show upstairs," she replies and tantalisingly adds, "But you can't come because you're a man."

But I can.

Seizing my chance, I suggest that one of my female

colleagues take me to have a look. It is a revelation. Immediately on entering the room, headgear is removed and I realise that many women wear false headpieces like huge scrunchies that lift their veils from underneath and add to the elegant poised look. It feels like I have walked into Aladdin's cave. If someone asks me to step on a magic carpet, I won't be a bit surprised.

They wear silk dresses and robes in jewelled colours, exquisite jewellery and make-up, particularly heavy kohl and the stuff they wear on the eyebrows to make them heavy and prominent. My dress is completely out of kilter, a pencil skirt and fitted jacket, but several of the women admire it. I have seen pictures of women at weddings and parties and they wear western clothes, often very skimpy but always colourful and exuberant.

My own flirty member of staff, Aliya, speaks very little English, but is able to say, "Sexy and beautiful," to my husband, while looking at me. Her ambition in life is to come to London with me, in order to learn English. I point out that this is not an option but I organise some English lessons for her in work time. She tells me that husband is not keen so she has not pursued the offer. Is he really making objections? Or is she just lazy and using him as an excuse? I will never know.

Although most Arab women cover their heads, not all wear the full abaya and niqab. There has been a recent flurry of emails about dress and the company lawyers have been particularly bothered. They seem to think they have a responsibility for upholding traditional Arab customs, although the Qatari doctors are less concerned as long as the medical practice is of a high standard. This is an extract from the first email:

I myself noted yesterday evening that two young female

doctors (not to mention nationality) among a group of
young doctors wore a short lab coat, well above the knees,
and under they wore tight stretch pants instead of the
normal loose pants.

I believe that I also spied one of the offending females, a beautiful medical student. The reply to the email from one of the Associate Directors of medical education is polite and thanks the lawyer for drawing everyone's attention to this important matter. (Incidentally he is the one with the pencil moustache, like the Tunbridge Wells bank manager). He goes on to describe how he takes aside miscreants and advises them accordingly. His email describes this:

But it seems they are still not aware of the seriousness of
this issue and deviate! I will take care of that personally by
directly advising them in a general quiet way (as we do not
advise such critical issues to be disclosed to them or dealt
by public either directly or indirectly).

This tempered message is not to the lawyer's satisfaction. He is not happy with a "general quiet way" but wants a policy that is clearly articulated, with sanctions. Moreover when he is presented with the existing policy, it isn't good enough.

There are clear loopholes in the policy attached:
a - it does not tell about the specifications, and dimensions
nor the colour. Is it allowed that every resident or doctor
shall decide for him/herself how his apparel should look
like?
b - it does not take into account, or even mention, the
traditions and customs of the local (dominant)Arabic

population in what is acceptable and what is not, instead, reference is made to 'multicultural patient population', and even no attempt is made to illegalize what is offensive or unacceptable to a patient's culture. I do not think that it will be acceptable for any culture that a female doctor shall attend duty wearing tight stretch pants under a short lab coat!

By now, several people have entered the fray and the responses are coming thick and fast. A dress code committee is suggested but one of the commentators feels that we could be more measured and allow doctors to use their own judgement in matters of dress:

We are dealing with mature educated doctors who are culturally competent most of the time.

Such an opinion is apparently completely unacceptable and merits the response:

The fact that we are dealing with mature doctors is not a justification that we allow them to be dressed the way they like. I have seen myself dresses which are off the beaten track and need to be checked and, irrespectively, we have to have that kind of regulation in place, before we hear and read criticism from the community and the media.

Criticism from the media is always a worry, in particular from the Arab press who are often highly critical of the hospital, especially when westerners are perceived not to be conforming to Arab ways such as dressing "off the beaten track" – potentially a major concern. However our measured correspondent has an answer – we must engage stakeholders, form a focus group, brainstorm the issue and most of all, we must be scientific about this:

Although you disagree with everything I said (you are entitled to your personal opinion) I agree with you though on one comment which relates to culture and public opinion and the image of our corporation. Don't forget that we deal here with a cohort of staff from multicultural backgrounds and proudly we respect cultural differences as long as decency is the rule. Instead of keep talking about it on the net or, as you said, in the media (although no one has seen that) ... we need a committee from stakeholders ... from both genders and from different backgrounds, starting with a focus group to brainstorm this issue and agree or disagree on a professional basis Then higher authority will approve a detailed policy and get committed to provide the needed resources and each team will be responsible to implement and monitor feedback and remediate. That's how we in Medical Education function USING A SCIENCE BASED APPROACH without intimidation or threats in a supportive professional environment.

You will note that all this will happen in a supportive non-threatening environment, but this is not good enough for the lawyers, who respond:

I think we are now coming to an agreement that it is necessary to have a corporate dress code for all classes of physicians (Albeit some innuendos in your message!). All organized hospitals have such a policy.

He also makes the legal point that without a policy we can't punish anyone and drifts into Latin in case anyone has missed his point:

Please note that we may not oblige an employee to a certain type of dress, or hold him/her accountable for violation unless we have in place a bylaw or policy prescribing the requirements for such dress code, 'no punishment except in accordance with the law' (nulla poena sine lege).

It is still running with multiple correspondents and diverse ideas. A query is raised about wearing a thobe and ghutra underneath the white coat and finally Lionel can hold back no longer. He points out that the white coats are filthy, are worn outside in the dusty desert and maybe infection control might play a part in this debate. No one is interested. We simply revert to concerns over young women wearing tight trousers. Still, following the emails brightens up my day. I wonder what they think of the hoots of laughter emanating from my office.

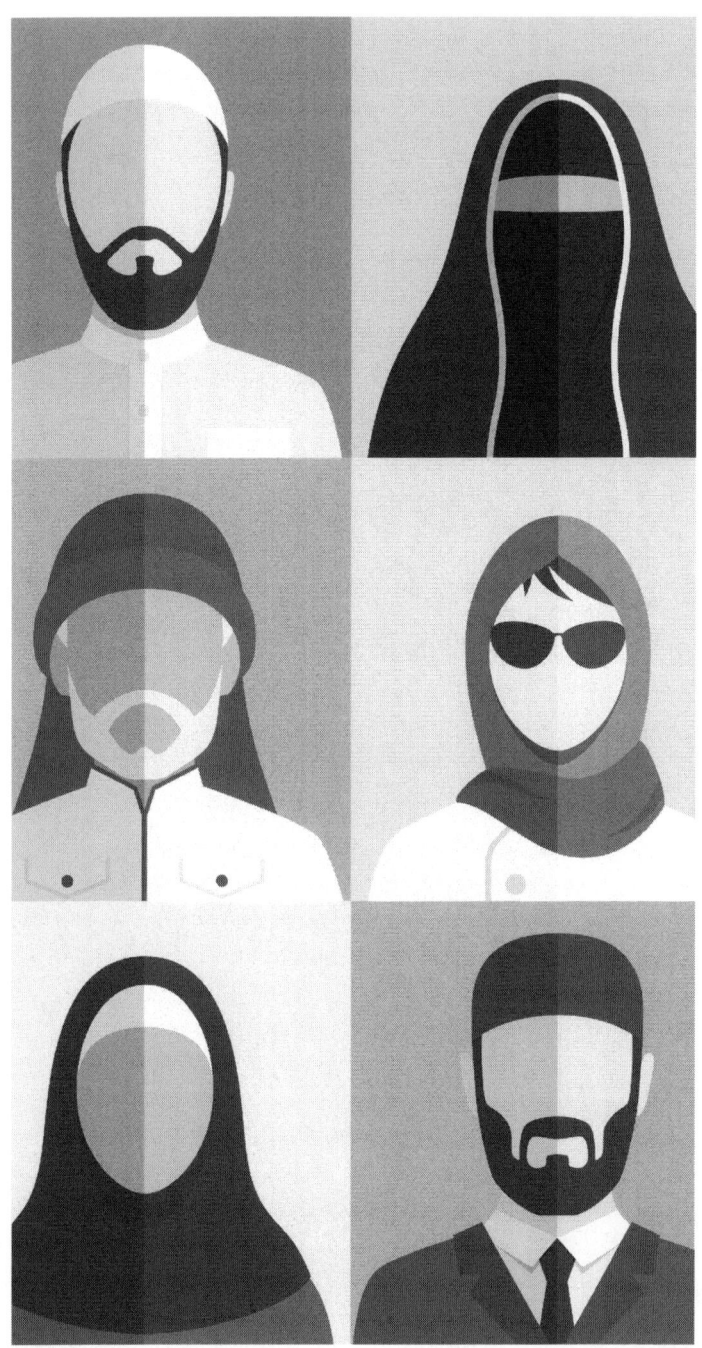

9

RAMADAN

We've had a bit of a false start. We were invited to Break Fast, known as *Iftar*, with some Muslim friends on Tuesday evening. But then the night before, it was all changed. Ramadan would start on the Wednesday and why? Because the moon committee had not sighted the new crescent moon. Now we Brits know about such things simply because we are aware of tides from an early age and tides are governed by the moon. Tide tables are published at least a year in advance and are remarkably accurate, so why can't these desert dwellers who live in a scientific age, predict the first day of Ramadan?

Admittedly we couldn't see the new moon either, but then we aren't the experts. Apparently one year there was a disagreement between two adjacent Arab nations and the timing of Ramadan was different as a consequence. We ask colleagues when Ramadan will start and these highly educated doctors start consulting almanacs, stroking their beards and discussing the response. Lionel witnesses three of his Arab colleagues talking for half an hour about the likely timing of Eid al Fitr, which is the holiday following Ramadan. A few days public holiday are granted but no one can predict how many and we have to wait for the Emiri decree, which is conveniently announced the day before.

An added complication is that this is extra holiday and not part of the annual leave allowance. How wonderful, you may think, except that if you take leave either side of Eid then the Eid days count as annual leave too! I could make a facetious comment about courtiers made of cards painting roses red because the Red Queen is due, except I've been given a beautiful long-stemmed rose that has been meticulously dyed so that all the petals are different colours of the rainbow, not to mention the twenty-four carat gold plated rose which was also a gift. We really are living through the looking glass.

Everyone fasts from just before the sunrise call to prayer, currently at about 3.30am, until Iftar at 6.30pm. They eat and drink nothing, not even a glass of water, during these hours. Work time has changed to 8am to 1pm for Muslims only. Any public display of food or drink consumption is frowned upon and until recently was an offence punishable by law. Lionel and I join in and fast on the first day, while quietly drinking water behind closed doors. I am determinedly carrying on throughout the holy month except I still drink water during the day and indulge in a hearty breakfast when I get up, not in the middle of the night.

Children as young as seven go into training, gradually increasing their hours of fasting and by the age of ten they are expected to fast like adults. The whole family will be awake to share the 3am meal (*Suhoor*). Of course a lot of sleeping is done in shifts, early morning and afternoon. Feasting goes on through the night and extravagant Suhoor buffets in the large hotels continue from 9pm until 2am the next morning. While Lionel and I are wasting away (well a few pounds lighter anyway), the radio gives tips on how not to gain weight in Ramadan, but though we listen for it no one tells us when the shops will be open.

Supermarkets are usually open during the day but opening hours of everywhere else are completely random with no indication of opening times on their doors. We presume the malls are buzzing into the early hours but we are disinclined to venture out then, not least because we have to do a full day's work the next day. There is no ambiguity over the sale of alcohol: it is expressly forbidden during Ramadan.

The first day of Ramadan sees an increase in accidents. Apart from numerous bumps and collisions, someone drives his Land Cruiser off the road ploughing into three workers who are resting on the grass verge and killing all three, while two labourers fall off high-rise buildings on which they are working. To a medic, it does beg the question as to whether the perpetrators of these horrific accidents were hypoglycaemic at the time. Other health risks include an increasing incidence of kidney stones during Ramadan, due to the intense dehydration inflicted on the faithful.

Two weeks in and the number of violent deaths admitted via the hospital has risen to twenty-two. The chief executive of one of the hospitals, a feisty African-American woman, remarked, "It's becoming like district Chicago round here!"

Stabbings and shootings are not unusual. In spite of this being a holy month, feasting and fights carry on into the night, out in the desert mainly, among opposing tribes.

Even the sophisticated, western-educated Arabs are tribal and our urbane Arab colleagues talk about the poetry wars that have lasted several generations. A cardiologist and a thoracic surgeon each come from notable families who have been at loggerheads for generations in a dispute as to who writes the best poetry. The two doctors often clash over clinical matters but it is their own poetry which really fuels enmity between them. And they are deadly serious.

Muslims may work from 8am to 1pm but we infidels have to put in the usual hours. It works quite well in practice, with meetings in the morning and catch-up time in the afternoon. Clinical staff might work slightly reduced hours but the patients keep coming, so the work goes on. It is tough for those operating or working in the Emergency Department, where there is no respite and no food or drink. The newspapers give helpful tips on how to deal with Ramadan, including reminders of the rules, which include:

No sexual intercourse with one's spouse.
No intentional emission of sperm unless asleep (followed by a remark about the perils of masturbation.)
Menstrual blood automatically breaks fast (but you have to make up the fast day when the period is over).
No swallowing blood from a nose bleed or it breaks fast.
No donating blood unless in dire emergency.

There are a few more seemingly incongruous rules such as not being allowed to induce vomiting in oneself. Unless you are at Roman feast and are handed a feather, or are a mistaken bulimic trying to vomit on an empty stomach, why would you? All the above can be done during the dark, except presumably intercourse with anyone other than one's spouse is still prohibited and masturbation is apparently still not acceptable, even by moonlight.

The month is designated as holy and alms-giving is encouraged. Good deeds are performed, such as taking Iftar to elderly people and breaking fast with them. Customer loyalty points can be traded in and given to charity and there are messages of generosity and tales of beneficence daily in the newspapers. A particularly charming story is that of *Garangao*, which is a children's tradition practised on the fourteenth day of Ramadan. The children dress up in traditional costume and sing a traditional song while onlookers ply them with nuts and sweets.

Alternatively the children might knock on doors and sing to the householder, who rewards them with goodies. One of my (Muslim, but non-local) colleagues suggested inviting the hospital teams to Iftar in one of the hotels as a way of thanking them for their efforts in an important project. I thought it was a great idea and consulted a senior Qatari, who agreed with the premise but advised, "The Qataris will not come as it is a time for families in this part of the Gulf."

Meanwhile we have taken to gazing at the moon in order to gauge progress. It is definitely starting to wane and the prospect of eating during daylight and our forthcoming holiday becomes increasingly tantalising.

Ramadan kareem (Blessed Ramadan) to all.

10

BUILDING BRIDGES

he Arabs want to embrace western medicine. They understand it in terms of the science and technical advances but in their own milieu they tend to revert to cultural norms. So although there is ostensibly a willingness to embrace teamwork across the professions, in practice the hospitals are still very hierarchical. This perpetuates a blame culture where mistakes are hidden, complaints are ignored and patient care is inevitably compromised. Not that we are perfect in the western world: we too have a long way to go.

One of the problems in HMC had been a disconnection between administration in the corporate offices and the clinical staff in the hospitals. Because of my strong clinical background I am able to build bridges between the two. The problem is how to get the messages across those bridges. I decide that we need a series of conferences or workshops where we can share ideas, discuss international research and together improve the systems underpinning patient care in our hospitals.

My slowly slowly, *shwai shwai* approach is working. The groundwork in reaching out to the hospitals across the country has been worthwhile. In terms of getting the doctors on side, I am pushing against an open door.

The corporate view is to engage some experts from out of town, somewhere convenient like London or New York. We have already done some work with the Harvard Business School, who have been fantastic, but only a small number of senior clinicians could be included in such an approach. My view is that we need to tap into the considerable expertise of our own doctors.

Moreover, I am not going to be there forever and I want to overcome the passive resistance and that learned helplessness that we all encounter. I want to cede control to the locals, to give them self-belief, to stop the constant blaming of the administration and encourage autonomy with inclusivity. Less of, "I'm the doctor and I know best," and more of, "We are a team. Let's work together to do the best for our patient."

So we invite every single consultant in the country to attend one of a series of one-day workshops in Doha. I will have the opportunity to meet each one individually, and to reinforce how much they are valued by me and the organisation. They will all have the opportunity to air their views.

It is a gamble and a risk. We wonder if they'll turn up: they do. We even have to put on extra days to accommodate them all. By giving everyone large easy-to-read name badges, I am also able to pretend that I know all their names, all six hundred of them.

I arrive after the usual battle through the traffic, draw up at the grand entrance and simply get out of the car, leaving my key in the ignition. I am greeted by, "Good morning ma'am" as I walk into the hotel. My car is valet parked and retrieved for me at the end of the day. When I arrive at the workshop venue, my completely veiled member of staff embraces me warmly, comments approvingly on my clothes, then presents me with a bunch of fresh flowers.

There are fifty senior doctors attending each day and I wander round the tables greeting people and chatting. Everyone is very warm and they all want to talk.

Discussion between lectures is vigorous and there are some great ideas around leadership and clinical practice. In the interests of inclusivity and breaking down barriers, I have invited the corporation's senior lawyer to one of the sessions, thinking that it will give him some insight into our medical values. We are doing much work currently on patient safety and on promoting a 'No Blame' culture. Our Sudanese lawyer with his British degrees is a confrontational man, as evidenced by his correspondence on dress code.

When he expresses concern that there is no rigorous punishment for doctors who have made mistakes, the response from one of the Qatari surgeons is voluble and emphatic in the extreme. With thobe and ghutra flying, he is on his feet shouting at the lawyer, who returns in kind.

"What does he know about medicine? He would put us all in jail for a simple mistake," pronounces the surgeon.

"Doctors think they are gods. He only operates for money like a typical plastic surgeon. The country needs lawyers like me to keep these doctors under control!" comes the swift riposte.

The insults are explicit. At one point the surgeon asks me, "Why is this man here?" to which I point out "He is my guest."

The exchange lasts several minutes before I am able, as chair, to restore order. Needless to say, the lawyer doesn't last the day and he is subsequently very peeved that I gave him no right of reply to the accusations against him. For good reason – it would have turned a skirmish into a full-blown battle, which none of us needed.

The gossip has already elevated the heated exchange to a stand-up fight. I am still not sure whether my reputation is enhanced or hindered by the incident.

If a session is in danger of over-running then I check with one of the senior Arabs to ensure that we are not running into prayer time. One day, the men decide to stay in the lecture room for prayers. One stands at the front with several others facing him and starts proceedings. They are at a slight angle to the geometry of the room so presumably someone knows the direction of Mecca. I also assume that they all kneel and touch the floor with their foreheads but I slip away quietly before they reach that stage.

Imagine such a scene at a UK conference. Here in Qatar, it is assumed everyone is religious and they all believe in God. These highly educated Arabs have no problem with the concept of evolution and have reconciled God and science in their minds and in their culture.

Occasionally I have interrupted someone at prayer in their office. Devotion is such a part of daily life that no one is surprised except us westerners. Many men display an area of thickened skin, a callus, on their foreheads from repeatedly touching the ground with their head when at prayer. A local who works in an adjacent department popped into my office recently with gifts from Mecca. He had just returned from pilgrimage and presented me with Arabian dates and holy water in a tacky plastic urn. He instructed me to drink it and pray. I was grateful and very touched, but can you imagine such a scenario at home? Not for the first time, I find myself musing that we are living in a modern world with a medieval mindset: but then the date here is 1450, so perhaps that makes sense.

The Emir publicly prayed for rain last week and this week we had a deluge. Since drainage is not a strong suit out here, the roads are consequently flooded and the accident rate is even higher than usual. No doubt the prayers are part of a long-standing ritual but I am sure many will believe that the rain was due to the Royal intervention.

Still, through my worries, the unexpected squabbles, and expected prayers, several people compliment me on the workshops, usually along the lines of, "I didn't want to come, but it has been good."

One neonatologist beckons me over to her table.

"I prayed to Allah that this would not be a waste of my time," she said. "Eight precious hours away from my patients is too much."

I looked into her eyes and waited.

She continued: "Allah answered my prayer. I have learned a lot today so I thank you."

Now I can smile and reply, "And thank you for being such an engaging participant."

The workshops are well received, my team is very supportive and well organised, and the hotel does well, with excellent food and facilities.

My personal learning is greatly enhanced by a camel conversation with two Arab doctors who confirm my suspicions that camels are supercilious, stubborn creatures.

They can survive for seven days in the desert without food or water but if they don't like you, they won't budge an inch. On the other hand, get it right and a camel will be loyal for life.

11

A BOOST IN THE BOOZE RATION

What a treat! An extra day's leave because the Emir is handing over to the Heir Apparent. This is a momentous occasion and unusual in these parts where new leaders are often the result of a coup, so a peaceful, planned handover done with wisdom and rejoicing is a joy to behold. In true Arab fashion, however, no one knew about this national day of celebration until 6pm the evening before, when the phone lines started buzzing and the text messages flew.

The stress of cancelling out-patients, elective theatre lists, job interviews and so on the evening before has cancelled out the holiday before it even begins. We did wonder whether we should carry on as usual, since we are a group of hospitals, but the message is clear – we should be seen to be celebrating. Anyway, the patients understand and don't turn up for their appointments. Lionel challenges the decision to cancel elective cardiac surgery on ethical grounds but the surgeons have no such compunction and lists are cancelled.

We watch proceedings on television and even though the commentary is in Arabic, it is pretty obvious that comparisons are being made between this Royal family and our own.

The new Emir and his father greet a long line of loyal subjects all paying their respects. They either shake hands, kiss the Emir on his shoulder or rub noses. We wonder how they know. What if you expect a nose rub but don't get one? Would the Emir think you were being too familiar?

One of our colleagues, who received the phone call to attend the ceremony, explains that there is a protocol, which is explained as you stand in line. He proudly shows us pictures of himself, in ceremonial black robe over his thobe, standing next to the new Emir and Father Emir, as the outgoing Emir is now known. It is such a small country that everyone knows everyone and a paediatrician colleague explains that he has often been summoned by the Sheikha (first wife) to see one of their four offspring at a palace in the desert.

There are two wives and the papers describe wife number one as an arranged marriage and wife number two as a love match. How do they know, I wonder?

Speculation in the hospital about the changes has been rife for weeks. There were rumours of our managing director becoming Minister for Health, bets were on who might replace her, talk was of who might fall if there was a change of regime. The colloquial term is *being put on a plane*, which in fact is entirely accurate as that is precisely what happens to people out of favour.

We laugh and quietly ensure that our money is sent home regularly, particularly Lionel's. This is another reason to have my own bank account. If he died suddenly, Sharia law would endow his estate to a male relative, probably to his eldest son, which would be fine, but if it were to be Lionel's brother in Canada that might be less straightforward. Without my own personal money I could be left temporarily destitute in an Arab country. If I died there would be no problem – everything would be Lionel's, obviously!

So in spite of the glitz and bling, the talk of a Knowledge Economy, and with education and health at the centre of government policy, there is still the sense of living in a Medieval world where the king is omnipotent and the courtiers fuss and bluster as they curry favour.

The term 'bank holiday' is, of course, a misnomer. The banks didn't close, or at least not the ones in the glossiest shopping malls.

On national days such as this, everyone drives down to the corniche, which is a beautiful road hugging the coast, lined with palm trees and providing spectacular views over the bay with its mixture of fabulous high-rise buildings, mosques, the wonderful Islamic museum and exquisitely lit dhows, gently floating by in the water.

The Royal family, like our own, walk among the crowds, talking and shaking hands with their subjects and there are military displays of soldiers on camels and horses. A traditional sword dance is *de rigeur* where the choreography never seems quite right, adding a certain frisson that someone might accidentally lose their head.

The patriotism of our new country infects us and we are almost homesick, but rally and decide to celebrate instead. So there is anticipation in our household as we await the arrival of one of Her Majesty's warships, *HMS DRAGON*. We know the Captain; in fact Lionel has been in correspondence with him but since they are on an operational mission, somewhat covertly.

I am naïve enough to be worrying about pirates as they pass through the Straits of Hormuse but as Lionel cogently points out, they are in the most advanced warship in the world so any pirates messing with them would definitely come off worse.

There is a certain sense of patriotism which rises to the fore, knowing that one of our ships is in port and as we approach the docks, we can see the distinctive grey radar tower above the assembled cargo ships and rust buckets alongside. Getting near her is more difficult. First we approach the dock gate, announce ourselves and confidently inform the guard that he has our names and that we are expected aboard the warship.

"No," comes the unambiguous response, accompanied by a desultory wave towards a building advertising itself as Dockyard Passes.

Nice try, except it is closed – so we drive round and find another entrance to the docks. This time we find a guard with a list, but our names are apparently not there. Lionel helpfully offers to look himself and is dismayed to find it all in Arabic. So all the westerners' names have been translated into Arabic and who knows what Chinese whispers have ensued. Suddenly there is a triumphant shout from the guard who has been quietly perusing his list under the shade of a tree. We have been found and we are in.

The ship is seriously impressive with big guns and missile launchers. The crew are unmistakeably British, particularly the officers in their white shorts and long white socks. On paper this always sounds quite ridiculous but somehow in the flesh, it works.

Lionel is completely at home on a warship and I find myself feeling very safe. I am also surprised that I feel an immense pride in our maritime nation, still sailing the seas and if not exactly ruling the waves, pretty close. We are given a personal tour of the ship and its helicopters and the impressive fast boat that can be lowered into the water within minutes, fully laden with marines and their weapons. The ship's company are all heading off to the rugby club and after weeks at sea, are ready for some relaxation.

Sadly for the Commonwealth sailors without British passports, this is not to be. Immigration are being tricky and refusing entry into the country because of an erroneous belief that someone with an African or Caribbean background would want to jump ship.

We invite the captain and his officers to a party at our house and are delighted when the whole wardroom accepts. Planning involves a meeting with the caterers but we think it judicious not to have them turn up at the same time as the cockroach exterminators. Large evil-looking cockroaches have occasionally been seen in the courtyard and we discover they enjoy living under the plant pots. The pest men come and spray noxious substances in the drains and under the plants. The vegetation doesn't suffer but thankfully the bugs do. They would be unwelcome guests at our party.

All is set for the evening and we have a good mix of local guests who have arrived by the time a minibus full of naval officers shows up. The Captain and our good friend Richard, who has flown out for the occasion, are already with us, fuelled up by Lionel's very dry martinis.

Our sixty or so guests mingle around the house and courtyard, which look amazing. We have a bar on the terrace while white-jacketed waiters move through the guests, deftly dispensing drinks. Two chefs resplendent in tall hats are ready next to their cooking stations. Red-and-white tablecloths cover the cocktail tables and the Royal Naval theme is intensified by hanging a large white ensign and Lionel's admiral's flag from the garage roof.

Scattered candles in Arabian lanterns bathe it all in a soft muted light. There is a chicken schwarma station, which is similar to a donner kebab. It is an Arabic dish, consisting of whole boned chickens that are packed together, skewered, flavoured with garlic, lemon and spices and then slowly spit-roasted. It smells and tastes delicious served in flat bread with salad. For the red meat eaters we have roast beef cut into thick slices and served in crusty baguettes.

The wine and beers are flowing and people are keen to sample the food, but first we have very brief speeches and I play *Rule Britannia* on my saxophone.

Everyone joins in and the call to prayer is completely obliterated by a rousing rendition from the assembled partygoers. We all feel intensely patriotic, while the staff give us that look of utter incredulity which says *You British are all completely mad.*

Incidentally, another urban myth has been dispelled, namely that one's allowance for alcohol is related to salary. A new myth has replaced it, that the quota is related to previous consumption. So we are unsurprised that following the visit of *HMS DRAGON*, our allowance for booze has just risen exponentially.

The warship has sailed and it is the weekend. The day is dull and overcast so everyone in Doha heads to the beach, including us. We arrive early afternoon after a long drive down the deserted four-lane motorway, surrounded by desert, scrubland and a few small oases of verdant trees. As we are near the sea we wonder if there are underground streams irrigating this vegetation. Our first attempt to find the beach fails and we almost head off into a wadi, where we would almost certainly have become stuck … but when in doubt, phone a friend.

She helpfully directs us back to the track where we encounter a posse of Land Cruisers heading off into nowhere. We follow in the usual random fashion, with everyone overtaking to left and right, until we reach the car park, where everyone alights and starts unpacking.

The sand is white and fine and the turquoise sea would be inviting but the clouds are grey and ominous-looking, so in spite of the high temperature a swim doesn't appeal. We elect instead to go for a long walk along the deserted beach, past the turtle nests, marked and protected, and watch the wading birds at the water's edge.

Ahead there is not a person in sight. In the far distance we can just make out the flares from the gas-fields, where all the wealth is created; the monotony of the landscape is punctuated by serried lines of electricity pylons marching across the desert to feed the city.

Energy conservation is not a concern out here. Petrol is dirt cheap and the skyscrapers downtown blaze with splendid light displays, while air-conditioning blasts away at full pelt. In the winter, there are outside heaters. Forget any idea of limiting plastic bag use: our supermarket purchases are packed by a helpful worker who uses three to our one and recycling is non-existent. Sadly some of these non-biodegradable items have found their way to this otherwise unspoilt and beautiful beach.

On our return, the scene on the beach has magnified. It is packed with families and groups of lads all making camp and barbecuing and from a distance the scene is reminiscent of an English beach. However, as we get closer the differences become apparent. A large carpet is *de rigeur*, with small tents for shade, barbecues in different stages of construction and an enormous amount of paraphernalia in the guise of foldaway chairs, tables and elaborately decorated shisha pipes. There is a strong smell of chargrilled meat mingled with the sweet aroma of the pipe.

Meanwhile the sea is heaving with bodies and one lone power boat, whose driver is cruising through the swimmers at speed while blasting out loud music. Everyone is ignoring him so eventually he gives up and roars away. Some of the picnickers have gone to lengths that would not disgrace the interval at Glyndebourne, although taking one's hubble-bubble pipe into the Sussex countryside would probably be viewed as eccentric.

There are western women wearing bikinis and many non-gulf Arabs in typical seaside attire. Thobes and abayas are less in evidence. A group of young Indian men are sitting cross-legged on their carpet, digging into large mounds of rice and vegetables which are placed in the middle of the circle. They are using their fingers and bread to scoop up the food and invite me to join them. Naturally I decline and Lionel notices that he didn't seem to be included in the invitation.

There are several such groups. They are likely to be migrant workers from the Industrial City that we have seen from a distance or from the massive number of construction projects in evidence all over the country.

Returning to work after the weekend, everyone remarked on the good weather. Gloomy overcast days are welcomed and when it rains they all take sick days and rush off into the desert, though Lionel and I still can't fathom the reason.

Winter is upon us and it feels cold. The temperature hasn't dropped into single figures but we are all wearing wool in order to feel cosy. The men have gone into brown woollen winter thobes with embroidered ghutras in shades of cream-coloured fine wool. They still wear sandals displaying horrible horny feet and toes. There is no doubt that the Arab dress is elegant, but the feet let them down.

The abaya-clad women are wearing beautiful shawls and I now know who buys those extremely expensive cashmere stoles seen in posh Italian shops; rich Arab ladies of course.

The Emergency Department is busy because it is the camping season. It gets bitterly cold at night yet they rush to the desert, erecting their tents then racing over the sand dunes in four-wheel drive vehicles, managing to inflict horrific injuries. The children are the most reckless. We encountered two little boys practising in the supermarket car park. They were riding together on a small quad bike, expertly spinning round the roundabout on two wheels. Yes they were good, but not invincible.

There is a fatalism in the Arab psyche which means that fathers drive cars with their tiny children nestled on their laps, mothers allow little ones to hang out of open windows while the car screeches round the impossible roundabouts, and no one wears a seat belt let alone straps a child into a car seat. It is all the will of God; *in sh'Allah* has a lot to answer for.

Winter for me is my birthday and although Muslims do not celebrate such events, they like to celebrate ours, so I am taken out to lunch by my team, who are a multi-cultural bunch of differing nationalities and religions. They all seem to be united by a love of fast food so I am treated to a feast of sizzling prawns, fried chicken and assorted kebabs, all of which are initially presented on menu cards where every dish's photo looks a particularly unappetising shade of orange.

The seating arrangements are very specific. We have to be in a secluded booth so that the niqab wearer is positioned with her back to the restaurant. She is happy to expose her face to us, the close team, as she eats, but often such attire enforces the wearer to discreetly lift her veil as she pops food into her mouth without exposing her features.

Excruciatingly, the restaurant staff sing me "Happy Birthday" and carrot cake is produced with a candle.

Then the most amazing cake, fashioned like a Louis Vuitton handbag, is produced and distributed to the whole corridor on our return to work.

12

FUNERAL ETIQUETTE

The mother of two of our colleagues has died. Funerals in Qatar happen very soon after death, followed by a week of official mourning when people go to pay their respects to the bereaved family. Businesses put huge advertisements in the newspaper extending their condolences to bereaved members of staff. The more important the employee, the more column inches there are. In our case, an email was sent to all staff, commiserating with the brothers.

The men organise a *majilis*, a gathering of the tribal elders and other invited men only, which is held in a large tent near to the house. It would have been inappropriate for me, a woman, to go so I enquire about the correct protocol. Apparently women go to see the female relatives in the deceased's house, so off I go with several other non-western members of staff. The plan is to go in convoy because only Maryam, one of the secretaries, knows the way, although it turns out that her knowledge is sketchy. Plans are always vague and timing is dreadful. Two of us are being driven by Aliya, my niqab-wearing member of staff, in her large Land Cruiser. That in itself is an experience not to be missed.

First we have to wait for Maryam. We loiter at the front of the main general hospital adjacent to our headquarters: it is the usual melee of cars, taxis and ambulances accompanied by a cacophony of horns honking for no obvious reason.

We drive around a few times until we spy a free parking slot. Aliya's driving technique is a wonder to behold.

"I can't park," she confides and proceeds to lower her window and summon the security man. "Move that bollard for me," she instructs, whereupon he does so and we simply drive into the slot alongside the curb. Things get tricky when the pristine white Rolls Royce in front starts to manoeuvre backwards, indicating that Aliya should do likewise.

Cars have enormous prestige out here and undoubtedly the young Arab in his roller is not only wealthy but well-connected. Luckily no scrapes happen and we all drive away intact. The journey is frightening. We don't drive in convoy but communicate by mobile phone, glibly weaving between lanes and cutting up other motorists as we go.

The car's interior is decorated in true Arab style. The headrests still sport the original plastic factory wrapping, which is a sign of a new car even if it is several years old. It fools no one but they all persist in doing it. Extras include dangling worry beads, frilly and furry cushions on the back seats and a bottle of Oud perfume with which we are liberally sprayed so that we arrive smelling like a dodgy bazaar.

As we near our destination we see Arabic signs to it and arrive along with several other women. I am the only westerner and I am greeted like a long-lost friend by one of the sisters, who grasps my hand and kisses me numerous times on the cheek, muttering thanks as she does so. We are ushered into a large reception room and offered tea in exquisite glass cups, served by the Filipina maids. There is a recording of verses from the Qur'an being played in the background in an incessant loop.

We all sit on chairs and sofas placed around the edge of the room and chat quietly. Since my Arabic is non-existent there is little I can say till I discover that one of the nieces speaks good English, so I engage her in conversation. She is a delightful teenager who wants to be an engineer so we have a good chat before a suitable moment comes for us to leave. Again the thanks are profuse and we leave as an elegant lady in a flowing abaya steps out of her Porsche and trips across the scrub to the front door.

I think no more about it until one of the brothers tells me how appreciated my gesture has been, particularly that I bothered to speak to one of the nieces. This impression is reiterated when one of the wives tells me that the family has been talking about my visit for days. What do I mean by *one of the wives*? I simply mean the wife of one of the brothers. However, translating the family set-up for me as we left the deceased's house, I discovered that there are two wives and that the sisters who greeted us are in fact half-sisters but that the families run concurrently and the mourning of the first wife is shared equally across the family.

Multiple wives are becoming less common but still occur, especially in rich families. A western-educated doctor explains it to me. "Although men can marry foreigners, women cannot and anyway there's a dearth of men," she says. It all seems very strange to us, but maybe we are just not attuned to the cultural mores.

"Why not?" she says, explaining, "maybe the first wife couldn't have children or maybe she didn't like sex, so why shouldn't the man marry again?"

I have also heard that a career woman might marry a man as his second wife so that she can easily continue her career without worrying about domestic issues.

Meanwhile Lionel has a case of sexual harassment to deal with. It's not quite *droit de seigneur*, but pretty close: a senior Arab harassing a young foreign woman. What to do? First inclination is outrage and confrontation, but what would that achieve? A plane ticket home for us and the woman would be left with nobody to protect or help her. On reflection, she is safe and nothing has actually happened, so she is swiftly moved to another post and the whole business is quietly forgotten. We then learn that apartments downtown are often rented by rich Arabs as places to take their mistresses; usually they are foreign girls who enjoy the gifts bestowed. It all smacks of hypocrisy and our tacit approval can feel uncomfortable.

There is pervading fatalism. Everything is God's will and *in sh'Allah* punctuates every other sentence. It can be irritating for us who think that we should give the Deity a helping hand. Trying to instigate emergency procedures, for instance, can be an uphill task.

Fire is frightening, especially in a hospital filled with sick debilitated patients. Evacuation plans and rehearsals are common at home but what is the drill out here? Lionel is sitting in a lecture at his hospital when the fire alarm sounds. There is no test scheduled and the alarm is very loud, implying that the fire is genuine and very near. No one takes a blind bit of notice. There is no smoke and

Lionel, who as chief executive is ultimately responsible for safety in the hospital, leaves the lecture in order to investigate. It appears that the cause is the coffee machine outside the lecture theatre: it's steaming and triggering the alarm, so there's no real danger, but not yet proven either.

However he is perturbed to discover that in spite of alarms and flashing lights at the entrance to the hospital, people continue to wander in and out unchallenged. Nurses are arriving for duty and the security guards are ignoring the incoming stream of visitors and patients, seemingly walking into a building that's *on fire*. Everyone is completely oblivious to the possible danger. His secretary is calmly chatting on the phone so he asks her if she is requesting information about the fire. "No," she replies simply.

Fire alarms are not unusual in hospitals and staff do have a tendency to ignore them, but in a country where there was a major disaster due to fire less than a year ago, this attitude is surprising. Fire broke out in a new shopping mall and the consequence was several deaths, among them a number of children who were being looked after in a nursery sited within the building. The whole episode was related in graphic detail at the hospital's fire lecture, which I attended recently.

The errors were legion: fire doors were padlocked, there was no plan for evacuation of shoppers and staff, and people became trapped on the roof. The worst thing was that the nursery did not appear on the plans of the building. Mothers were screaming that their children were trapped, only to be told that there were no rooms on the plans in the location the mothers had indicated. When eventually the fire was brought under control and the firefighters, several of whom also lost their lives, broke into the nursery, they found all the children and their carers dead from smoke inhalation.

Are we simply mercenaries, taking the money and putting up with it all? There is an element of that and some of our Arab colleagues see Westerners in that guise. On the other hand, while we are certainly not missionaries, we like to think that we have something to offer and wish to impart that knowledge so that any positive change is sustainable. The argument then goes: well if you want change then you have to become accepted and trusted and that won't happen without some acceptance of cultural mores even if, superficially, they are anathema to you.

So we press on, extolling the good things, building relationships, trying not to be judgemental yet holding onto a moral compass of sorts.

13

A PYRRHIC VICTORY

I t is our second Christmas and we have been here sixteen months. By now I have managed to build a fiercely loyal team, not easy given the difficulties with recruitment.

Joramae is a gem. She is remarkably adept linguistically, having been born in the Philippines and brought up in Saudi Arabia. Hence she is bilingual in Arabic and English and speaks three Philippino dialects. She also has a pharmacy degree, remarkable emotional intelligence and knows everyone. She would be perfect as my assistant executive director but, because of the perverse labour laws, she cannot be promoted – so I am trawling the ex-pat head-hunters to find someone suitable.

Andrea fits the bill perfectly. She arrives and in a no-nonsense way gets to work with the Arabs in outlying hospitals. She builds up a good relationship with the plastic surgery team who then give her tips on how they might improve various bits of her anatomy. She is a good-looking woman who has no need of such work. The surgeons merely laugh and say, "Well if you change your mind, Miss Andrea, you know where we are." It is fascinating that they feel comfortable with making such personal observations. I seem to have escaped, but maybe they think I am beyond improvement.

Things are getting better. I am building up my team. Honeylet's replacement was poached by an unscrupulous colleague so for a while, I had no secretarial support. Joramae came to the rescue. She found a Filipino schoolteacher who had fallen out with his Qatari employers for unfathomable reasons. Nevertheless he was keen to stay in the Gulf and to bring his family over to live with him. His clammy handshake and tense expression revealed his nervousness when I interviewed him. He had no direct secretarial experience but was well educated and keen to learn so I took a risk. It paid off and he has proved a loyal and companionable worker.

Achieving even the smallest or most trivial thing here can take an amazing amount of time, effort and wheeling-and-dealing

There are masses of new hospital buildings under construction but somehow they never get finished. Meanwhile we are appointing new staff in droves and there is nowhere for them to work. The solution is obvious: send staff working in an adjacent building into a new block off-site, then move our admin staff into the vacated space.

Unsurprisingly no one wants to go. Possibly if plush new offices were on offer it would be different but sadly the reality is that this is a communal open-plan space off-site.

I have not been involved in the planning and anyway it isn't really my responsibility, but with the boss away and the incumbent statisticians deciding on a sit-in, I am called in to sort out the mess. Their diminutive professor is angry: diplomacy and tact seem the only solution. Keep him talking. He is originally from Turkey and as I extol the virtues of the Aegean coast, he starts to calm down. Eventually he agrees to move half his team.

It's a Pyrrhic victory since that still doesn't leave enough space for the incomers, our admin staff. This move is like a line of dominoes except they are falling haphazardly and there is no contingency plan. Actually it becomes increasingly apparent that there is no plan at all. From memory of the new offices, I sketch a floor plan on my flipchart and allocate a few desks and suddenly people are crowding into my office (luckily I am staying put) to see The Plan.

Not that they take any notice. It is first come, first served and still the statisticians are reluctant to leave and make way.

Meanwhile someone complains about the smelly carpets and then termites are discovered, so an army of painters, pest destroyers and cleaners appear among the complaining exiting statisticians and the newcomers bagging all the best desks. Anarchy doesn't even begin to describe the chaos.

I retreat to my own territory where Aliya is in melt-down. She isn't moving over there. The large, heavily made-up eyes are flashing above her niqab as she tries to explain that as an Arabic speaker she needs to be near me in order to converse with people in Arabic, thus helping my communication. This is a fair point except that she doesn't speak English, so her skills as an interpreter are somewhat limited.

However, my advice is always to choose your battles and I am unlikely to win this one so I capitulate but explain that she has to move desks. "No problem", is the reply and this time the eyes are smiling. She settles in next to my male secretary, bringing her assortment of trinkets, dates, boxes of Arabic sweets and other such useful paraphernalia on her desk.

By now things have calmed down over the road. The professor has gone on leave back to Istanbul and his staff have moved into their off-site offices, grumbling about the lack of parking. There's actually plenty of parking: they simply mean there are no named spaces and the new car park is built on European lines, which means that it is necessary to manoeuvre the car into a space rather than sweeping into the slot in one easy motion. Meanwhile the walls of the newly emptied space have been freshly painted … although there is now a hole on one wall where the termites were happily munching until the exterminators arrived.

Back in my corridor, I am surveying the scene when Aliya of the niqab comes in and tells me, with a combination of halting English and body language, that a senior Arab has passed by and is appalled that she, a local woman, is being made to sit opposite the gents' lavatory. This is an exaggeration since the gents is in fact across the corridor, down another and around a corner, but again, deciding that this is another battle to dodge, I arrange for her to go somewhere else, after much cajoling of other staff. Peace at last, except that she doesn't want to go there, but wishes to stay in the room with my secretary. Her solution is simple: she will nick someone else's desk, then they can face the lavatory. The unfortunate, putative lavatory gazer spends most of her time elsewhere (in a place where space is at a premium, one might ask why she is allowed the luxury of two desks, but the answers would be unbelievably opaque) so I agree to the niqab-wearer's desk nicking plan.

Five minutes later my secretary sidles into my office and explains that he feels very uncomfortable sharing an office with a veiled Qatari lady.

"Don't worry," I assure him. "She might wear it but she isn't religious and she couldn't care less."

"But I am religious," he explains, "and it makes me uncomfortable. In fact I can't work there."

So now we have grumbling statisticians in their off-site open-plan office, but their professor has somehow kept a personal office on-site. Some of our staff have moved into the vacated offices but have used three of the spaces for large, unwieldy and unnecessary filing cabinets, so we still have too few desks and my male Muslim Filipino secretary is floating around trying to dodge the flirtatious niqab-wearer. The boss is back next week! Good to know that we start the New Year in good shape.

Lionel points out that the pinnacle of my career has turned into becoming an ex-pat overseer of multi-cultural office allocation, not unlike a medieval bazaar – as ever, back in the Middle Ages.

The addendum to this story is that the blustering fussy professor is subsequently accused of *cooking the books*. He is said to be creaming off research grants for his own personal use. Whether this is true or not, no one knows but he goes in a hurry. I last see him clearing out his office.
"I've resigned," he beams. "I'm on the plane back to Istanbul tomorrow."

Presumably he thinks it best not to argue his case.

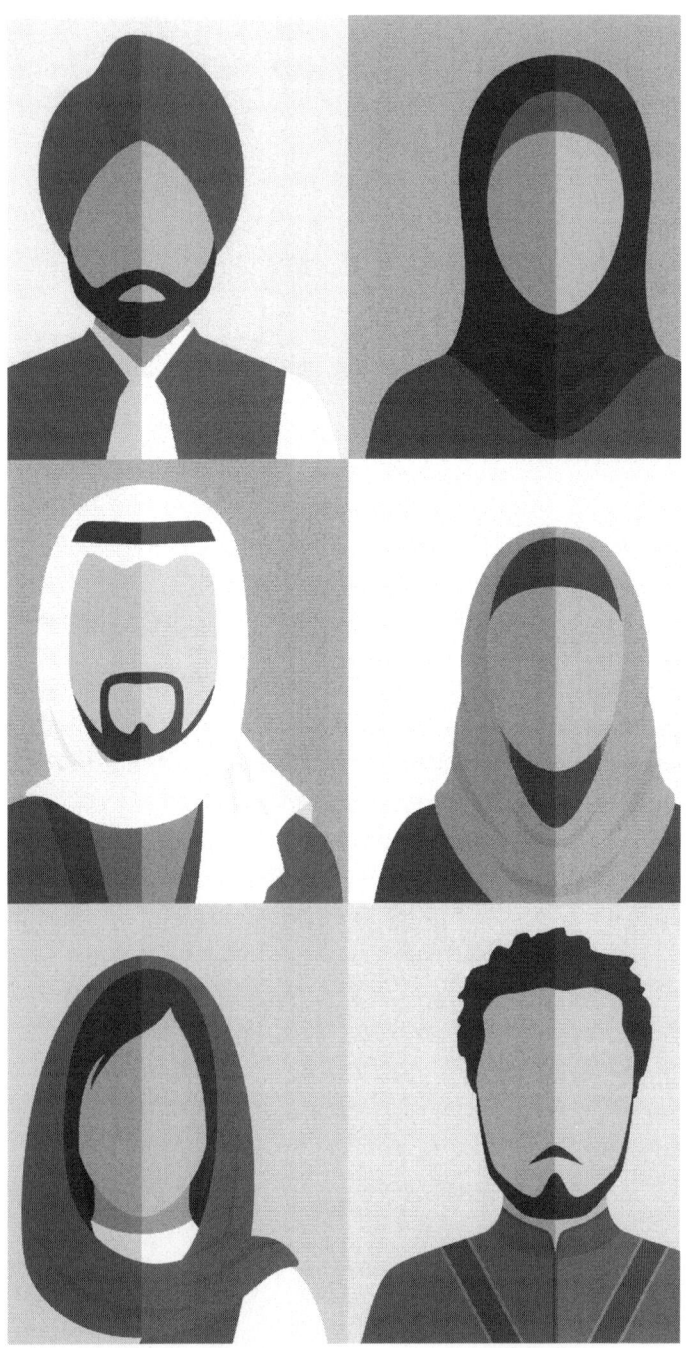

14

FOREIGN AFFAIRS

We keep a close eye on world events, and although the Middle East is in turmoil and friends in the UK worry about us, we reckon that Qatar is as safe as anywhere from threats of terrorism. Within the first few weeks of our arrival we experienced Arab diplomacy in the raw, while still ensconced in the Ritz Carlton hotel.

Our hotel was certainly in the thick of things. One week we had a world military conference and we couldn't move for military types dripping in medals and gold braid. Lionel pointed out that most countries in the world seem to have copied our basic design and elaborated on it. Increasing the bling factor was clearly a high priority in many states. There were numerous cars with diplomatic plates in the car park and alongside the usual array of Land Cruisers were a selection of cars painted a matt red colour, which designated the military police, but only in an Arab state would they be Porsches.

Last week it was the Syrian National Congress meeting, which was fascinating. As I write, President Assad of Syria is ravaging his country, civilians are being killed and the purpose of the congress was to choose the Opposition in exile, as a challenge to President Assad and his cronies.

We would read about events in the newspaper then recognise one of the opposition players having breakfast at an adjacent table. Security was increased and an x-ray machine installed at the hotel entrance into which bags were put while the guests walked through a sensor similar to those found at airports. Sitting at the desk behind the bag machine was a young Arab, intent on texting on his mobile phone and seemingly paying no attention whatsoever to the screen in front of him, while the punters passing through the sensor caused a series of bleeps that were received with a wry smile by the security guards ... who then did nothing.

The on-stage part of this important world event was closed to us but we were able to experience Arab diplomacy simply by sitting in the hotel lobby and watching. Groups of men would congregate (I counted only a handful of women) with much hugging and kissing on the cheeks. Conversation was loud and voluble and people would move between groups whereupon these tactile demonstrations would be repeated. Occasionally a couple or three would separate to sit and drink coffee before returning to the fray.

The noisiest times were in the evening after dinner and appeared to continue into the night judging by the loud telephone conversations emanating from our next-door neighbour's hotel room. Delegates wore a mixture of dress, some in thobes and varying head-dresses, but many were dressed in western style. Sheikhs were resplendent in long flowing robes with an outer black or brown robe expensively trimmed with gold. One of them was certainly eyeing me up with a lascivious smile, much to Lionel's discomfort (although I suspect Lionel was secretly wondering about the price of camels!).

Travelling between floors by lift was carefully controlled by having to insert your room card before pressing the button for a floor. This means that you are unable to visit another floor and during the Syrian National Congress, when the delegates' homeland is being ravaged by civil war, security might be expected to be on serious alert ... but no. The system was switched off so that anyone who managed to breach the security entering the hotel could then wander its corridors with impunity. Moreover as the delegates started to leave, their exact itineraries were posted in Arabic in the lobby for all to see. Thankfully there were no incidents or threats and the local press deemed the congress to have been an exceptional success.

Generally Doha is a great venue for large international meetings and the Qataris love to show off their city and its amenities. At HMC we are organising one such event. My role is not a major one so I can observe the conference with an objective eye.

Delegates from all over the Gulf are flocking to the conference centre, which is a splendid futuristic building with huge lobbies, grand lecture halls and more intimate wood-panelled areas for small group working. I drive past the university and follow the signs to the VIP parking. The uniformed security guard has a list but doesn't check me, simply handing over a VIP pass and directing me to the special car park. Lionel is less lucky and undergoes laborious checking procedures before being let through. Sometimes it helps to be a blonde western woman with a big smile.

The marble and steel central atrium is embraced by a huge sculpture of a spider, which is familiar since it once had pride of place in the turbine hall of Tate Modern. The delegates, numbering two thousand in total, scurry around below the eight legs, booking sessions, eating, drinking, greeting each other, while the American visitors move in packs shepherded by an important-looking man in a grey suit carrying a walkie-talkie.

I am scheduled to chair a few sessions so I find the right lecture theatre, make contact with the black-clad audio-visual technicians and greet the American expert who is to speak. But first we have the opening ceremony. As usual, very very important people (VVIPs) have designated seats in the front row, while simple VIPs have to be content with rows two or three. Inevitably the front row is a sea of white thobes and ghutras, with an occasional grey suit. I appear to have been forgotten, so my success with the VIP parking is short-lived.

I bump into a Qatari female consultant colleague who offers me a seat next to her, where we have a good vantage point of the great and good, most of whom she knows anyway. She is much younger than me and very beautiful, with heavily made-up eyes and fingers and wrists dripping with diamonds. I spy a hint of genuine Pucci print beneath her black abaya and the official photographer spends most of his time photographing us both together while ignoring important Arabs and American academics.

My subsequent sessions over the next two days go well, with excellent speakers from the United States who manage to engage the large audiences well in spite of the size of the venues. I control the questions and we keep to time, which is not always easy in this place since Arab questions have a strong tendency towards narrative and hence take ages before finally getting to the point.

The second day I bump into my new best friend again, in one of my sessions. She is wearing a new abaya, which is the customary black but adorned with lines of biker jacket studs along the sleeves and on the veil. She is wearing vertiginous heels and sporting a designer handbag. The effect is rock-chick meets punk meets the Middle East. She looks stunning and she knows it.

We are chatted up by a young man from a neighbouring country as we leave the lecture theatre. He wants to impress me because he thinks I might be important but he is mesmerised by her, especially when he discovers that she is a surgeon. She simply looks down her long aquiline nose at him and he visibly crumbles. He hasn't a chance.

Sitting on the organising committee for this event, I become painfully aware of the incipient chaos that underpins it. Yet somehow, amazingly it all goes smoothly, unlike an event two weeks earlier held at one of the five-star hotels, where the number of delegates had been severely underestimated and the pricing system for entrance added to the confusion.

There were three types of entrance fee: one that didn't include refreshments, one that did, and one that also included a *free* iPad. It was also possible to pay on the day so when, on the morning of the conference, hundreds of people turned up, the organiser decided to dispense with payment (it wasn't as if the organisation needed the money), vouchers for food were not issued and people were fighting over iPads. The food disappeared within minutes at the coffee break.

In the sessions there were crowds of nurses sitting at the back, eating picnics and taking photos, making a really good day of it but completely ignoring the speaker at the front. I suppose it is one way to earn continuing education points for the portfolio.

There is always an official dinner attached to these events to which we are invited. Such dinners can be turgid affairs, with non-alcoholic sticky drinks being served followed by enormous buffets, where the food is good but formulaic and conversation can be stilted without the lubricant of a couple of glasses of wine. The Americans seem to cope with this better than the Brits but then they think that we are all subclinical alcoholics anyway.

Unlikely though it might seem, there is a hospital here in Qatar, recently built by Emiri decree and staffed almost completely by Cubans. It is situated in the middle of the desert, surrounded by oil fields near the coast. I visited last week to meet the Chief Executive, who is Australian and the Medical Director, who is Cuban. The hospital itself is beautifully designed, with spacious wards containing single rooms, excellently equipped and surrounding a tranquil inner courtyard.

Although very contemporary, it has the peaceful air of the medieval hospital that I once visited in Florence. Apparently the Emir and Castro are good chums, which considering that Cuba is one of the longest and most successful Communist regimes and the Emir's is capitalist in the extreme, is somewhat incongruous. Still, they are both dictators of sorts so maybe they find something to chat about, even if only their shared love of deep-sea diving.

Visiting the Cuban hospital entailed a trip across country. This turned out to be the usual fraught journey. I had been warned that there were road works so when the diversions appeared I wasn't unduly worried. After one set of big red arrows, the signage ceased so I trundled on down increasing unlikely roads whereupon the track finally petered out and I was facing desert. The truth quickly dawned: this wasn't a diversion. It was the wrong way.

Turning round, I retraced my route and attempted to get back on track.

There are never any signs and I was forced to determine my direction of travel from the position of the sun. Except I couldn't see the sun from my car seat, so had to deduce its position from the shadows made by passing vehicles, in order to work out whether I was going in the right direction. All ended well when I found myself back on a decent road going west, so I assumed all was fine. It was worth the trip when I passed a random collection of tents with a corral containing camels and several groups of camels being exercised – a splendid evocative sight.

There was little traffic, a few goats by the side of the road, evidence of civilisation with telegraph poles and the like ... but no buildings. Because I knew there were no other highways going east to west, I couldn't possibly be lost and it felt like a big yet manageable adventure.

In fact I was so supremely confident that I managed to sail past the Cuban hospital and was forced to drive for several more kilometres before finding a way back on the other side of the dual carriageway.

The return journey was even more interesting. On the drive out, I had been so engrossed looking at shadows and I confess, feeling a bit smug at my navigational skills, that I had completely failed to notice the enormous fort, enclosed by thirty-foot crenelated walls interspersed with imposing gates. This fort covers several acres and houses the Emiri Guard, which is His Highness's personal guard. I had also managed to miss the various palaces and grand houses being built adjacent to the highway.

Not all palaces are so obvious. Lionel once sensibly stopped to answer his mobile phone by pulling off the road into a driveway. It said *Private* but there were no gates or guards. It could have been the entrance to one of the numerous compounds. His phone call was abruptly interrupted by an armed uniformed guard who had drawn alongside in his patrol vehicle, and aggressively asked if he had seen the sign.

"No," replied Lionel somewhat disingenuously.

"Your first fault. Give me your resident's permit, follow me in your car, then stay in the car," the uniformed officer commanded.

Some time later, presumably having made a few checks, he returned.

"Do you know where you are?"

"No," said Lionel.

"Your second fault," was the steely reply.

At this point, Lionel was estimating the price we might get for flogging the new furniture when he was deported, but the guard sent him away with a stern warning. This might be construed as a fair cop, except Lionel had no idea what the offence might have been. Looking at the map later, it became apparent: he had tried to break in to the Sheikha's palace i.e. the home of the Emir's most important wife.

Extraordinary things become commonplace. Yesterday evening, collapsing in front of the television, we found ourselves watching a Bollywood medical soap that had been dubbed into Arabic, when Immigration phoned Lionel to check whether one of his employees at the hospital was allowed to leave the country. Earlier that day, I had signed several memos giving permission for quite senior people to have exit permits.

Because Lionel's hospital is brand new, with well-appointed private rooms, the local VVIPs prefer it and he has to scurry around finding extra rooms for bodyguards, special nurses and other staff. The last VIP wanted no one to know that he was ill and Lionel had to carry on while pretending there were no armed guards or fleets of special Land Cruisers surrounding the hospital. It was a relief when the VIP was whisked away to London on the Emir's special flight.

This aeroplane is an Airbus fully equipped with a Critical Care Unit and inevitably, several of Lionel's senior consultants simply had to accompany the VIP. One of them was on-call but didn't see the need to inform anyone. There was some political fallout from that event as the Managing Director was furious that she hadn't been informed and blamed Lionel (who had been told not to tell anyone!). Astonishing that she didn't know. One of my Qatari colleagues remarked to me, "We are a small country. Abdulla sneezes in the souq and we all know by lunchtime."

Sometimes the politics are helpful as when a relative of the Minister was admitted to Lionel's hospital; the Minister called into Lionel's office for a chat. The next day the massive extension to Lionel's hospital was approved as a national priority with no regard to any previous plan or priority. Not all ministers are so obliging: another new hospital was ready to be opened when the Minister visited and didn't like the colour of the marble. All was delayed while the façade was changed to the Minister's taste. We are getting used to it and wouldn't be surprised if a white rabbit rushed past fiddling with his gloves and worrying about being late.

We were on a brief trip to London when my secretary phoned on my mobile and said that I needed to talk to Professor Matt urgently.

"Can you go to Cuba on an official mission?" Matt enquired. "No pressure but we need to know now."

"Of course," I replied. "I need to change a few arrangements but that's fine."

Three weeks later and we are due to fly to Havana in four days time. The official mission is to recruit staff for the Cuban hospital. There are three Arabs going: my surgeon friend Mustafa, another good friend –Wisam – who is a surgeon originally from Iraq, and Mohammed who is in charge of admin for the mission. Then there's Donald the Scottish obstetrician and me. The mission still hasn't been formally approved, the flights aren't booked and we have no visas for Cuba. We think that we are expected and allegedly we have hotel rooms booked in the Hotel Nacional. There is the usual Arabian chaos over the next two days: all flights seem to be full and the in-house travel office wash their hands of the arrangements, having initially suggested flying via Moscow or possibly Montreal. I elect to make my own way and at great expense (hopefully remunerated), decide to travel via Paris, stop for a night, then go out on the Air France flight to Havana. I use a UK bank card for this last leg of the journey, which prompts a call from the bank in England. They are suspicious of an individual flying from Paris to Havana, claiming to live in the Middle East and paying for the journey in Saudi riyals (I can't explain the latter either but that's how the website handled it). When I also thought about the fact that I had taken out 3,000 euros in cash, given to me in 200 euro notes, I reflected that I might well be suspected of some nefarious activity.

The reason for the cash is simple. Most credit cards won't work because of long-term US sanctions against Castro's regime. Eventually all paperwork, visas, remuneration and so on is sorted and I fly into Cuba where I am met by two delightful government officials who whisk me off to the hotel. There, I am met by Mohammed, whom I barely recognise without his traditional dress.

"Come and have a drink," he says. "What'll it be,

whisky or beer?"

A cold beer is very welcome and the tone is now set for the visit. We are going to enjoy ourselves.

Work starts in the old school, which is light and airy with shaded outdoor walkways surrounding gardens filled with tropical plants. A breeze blows through the open windows and ruffles the bougainvillea in the window boxes. We are treated to a brief history of the humanitarian work of the Cuban mission. It all started with relief work following Hurricane Mitch several years ago and the concept has continued with relief in various Latin American countries, and in Africa and Pakistan.

The *Commandant en Jefe*, as Fidel Castro is constantly referred to, offered his country's services to New Orleans following Hurricane Katrina but the offer was declined.

Pictures of Castro are everywhere: Fidel giving blood, Fidel meeting the Venezuelan president, Fidel rallying the troops. Pictures of the 'imprisoned five' abound: these are five Cubans who were interred on terrorist charges in United States gaols. Two have now been released but the others are serving concomitant life sentences. Whether they are guilty or not we are never told.

The journey from Havana through the countryside is a delight. Traffic is light and the 1950s cars painted in vibrant colours bash along with windows open and three abreast in the front bench seats. On closer inspection the Buick, Ford, Chevrolet and other marks are falling off, the tyres are worn and wings are missing, yet still the overall impression is of survivors clinging to their rich vibrant culture.

Music is everywhere. Even before the interviews, Mustafa, my surgeon friend, persuades our interpreter and our tea lady to break into song and dance. They need little persuasion and like most Cubans they have natural pitch and rhythm.

As our bus rolls through the countryside, we see people everywhere, walking, waiting at bus-stops, waiting at the level crossing. There is no obvious barrier but we stop as a train trundles past on a narrow-gauge railway track, like something out of a rather scruffy toytown. Havana itself is a mix of imposing statues, stately villas and colonial squares with glorious old Spanish buildings that are literally crumbling away, though thankfully some of the facades are now being restored with splendid results. When I accepted the job in Doha, I had little notion of what to expect but never imagined rubbing shoulders with such diverse regimes and people. Yet in spite of the different cultures and social norms, we all get on well as people. Living in a dictatorship is uncomfortable for those of us used to democratic systems, but people do cope. They have to … and they learn when to keep quiet.

We have over eighty candidates to interview over several days and we are informed of the numbers of doctors and technicians required, broken down by specialty. Candidates have arrived from all over Cuba and are staying in the school. We have a short-list that turns out to be complete fiction. As, one after the other, the hapless candidates are brought in, we realise that the organisation of the process is such that we have no idea who will walk through the door next.

Our first candidate, before we have got into our stride, says that she is an Immunologist. This doesn't tally with our list and her experience with x-rays and ultrasound is somewhat incongruous. We then realise that she has been claiming to be an Imaginologist. In my own radiology career, colleagues may have thought that I was imagining lesions on x-rays but at least I wasn't fraudulent, unlike our poor candidate who proudly boasted on her CV to be an expert in 'CT SCAM'.

Good English is a pre-requisite and in fact she gets through: others were less lucky. One poor woman is so nervous that she tries to run away and has to be persuaded by government officials to stay and return the next day. She has no English and is clearly unhappy at the prospect of being sent to a small desert country thousands of miles away. We don't accept her.

We have no notion of who might come next. We interview several Optometrists and Physiotherapists who come in random order. Our credentials, as a Radiologist and Obstetrician, are not ideal for this task but we warm to it. When the next candidate states that he is an English teacher, however, we decide that something is seriously wrong.

"No, it's fine," says Mohammed, "We need an English teacher in the hospital."

So he is appointed.

Although it is a completely random process, Donald, the Scottish professor. and I soon work out a system whereby we can decide on the best candidates. By the end of three days, we have finished while our Arab colleagues in the next room are still interviewing, inviting candidates to sing and occasionally popping in to see us for a chat – mid interview. They even try to help by inviting the government interpreter to come and work for us, causing much confusion.

On the final day we all sit down and discuss the results with the Cubans.

Professor Donald and I produce our list and are done within five minutes. The Arabs and Cubans deliberate for about two hours. It seems rude to leave, so Donald catches up on his emails while I try to engage in the discussion. The lists are pored over, swapped between parties, coffee is fetched, but nothing seems to happen. Certainly there are no decisions being made. Eventually I whisper to Donald:

"What are they doing?"

He looks up and replies laconically: "Don't know."

At which point I lose it and collapse in uncontrollable giggles.

Inevitably on a foreign mission there is time for relaxation and bonding with colleagues. The three Arabs have all been to Cuba before and are keen to show us the sights. We are treated to music and dancing with the elderly musicians who performed with the Buena Vista Social Club. The hotel where we are staying was one of the prime locations in pre-revolutionary Cuba and was much frequented by the Mafia.

The nightclub carries on the tradition of exuberant costumes, and excellent singing and dancing in a venue that feels like a speakeasy. The Mojitos are perfect and I am persuaded to smoke a large Havana cigar. I am way outside my comfort zone on the smoking front, what with hooker pipes in Arabia and cigars in Cuba, The first evening I comply, treating it as a bit of a dare, but I admit that the second evening, I rather enjoy it. There is something about the atmosphere in this extraordinary place that allows inhibitions to be shed.

The plan is to be taken by one of the (Qatari) embassy drivers out to a beach, have a swim and maybe some lunch. We arrive and two of the Arabs want to go to the rather tacky beach resort shopping centre. Parking the car is tricky as there is a gang of dodgy-looking men in sharp suits, with suspicious bulges under their jackets, directing us away from the car park. We then discover that the Angolan president is visiting with his bodyguards. Our driver points out our diplomatic plates and suddenly we are all best friends.

We find the beach but there is nowhere to change. The

Scot and I are unfazed, having spent our childhoods changing on cold windy beaches, under skimpy towels. However for an Arab this concept is too much to contemplate so we head off for lunch instead. The venue is a beautiful hotel overlooking a marina, and the tables are outside next to the water. Idyllic except that the hotel is full of western tourists and is not open to passing trade.

Our Arab colleagues simply have no understanding that we are being sent away. "But we have eaten here before and now we need lunch," they cry. Phone calls are made and suddenly we are made welcome.

The whole day has been a fascinating insight into the psyche of these rich Arabs who expect everything to happen as they wish it. The heartening thing was that our Cuban driver from the embassy escorted us to the lunch table then retreated, but was persuaded to stay and eat with us. We treated him: again, a good example of Arab generosity and hospitality.

Back in Qatar, Lionel and I take the opportunity of travelling more locally. However, travelling around the Gulf region is not always straightforward so, with an impending trip to the Sultanate of Oman, we scrutinise the website. This clearly advises obtaining our visas in advance, especially since we are British passport holders. The embassy website also helpfully includes a Google map, so we set off on a visa mission.

We have been here long enough to know that most maps are a waste of paper and sure enough, there is no embassy corresponding to the dot on the map. However, the sat nav indicates that we are in the Diplomatic District so, ever hopeful, we cruise around and find a different embassy, where we think we might get directions.

Lionel stops the car, walks through the embassy gate and disappears from view. It is only then that I ponder whether wandering into the Palestinian embassy is a good idea, especially when a guard appears from his hut and surveys me in the car, parked rather badly, with an expression of deep suspicion. I act very cool but breathe a sigh of relief when he ambles back into his guard house.

My equanimity is short-lived: he reappears with an AK 47 under his arm, pointed vaguely in my direction, presumably wondering whether a car bomb is about to explode from my position. Fortunately Lionel emerges from the gate, waves nonchalantly in the direction of the armed soldier and we go on our way.

"Did they tell you how to find the Omani embassy?" I ask.

"Hadn't got a clue," says Lionel.

Eventually we find it, in a completely different location of course. We ask for visas whereupon the official looks at our passports.

"But you are British," he says proudly.

"Well, yes, exactly," we reply, whereupon we are told to obtain the visas on arrival at the airport in Muscat. He clearly has no knowledge of the website instructions. We give up.

We are fortunate to have been granted multi-exit visas. Others are not so lucky. A Muslim colleague from the Philippines asked permission to travel to Mecca on pilgrimage, as she has done for the last five years. Her flight was at midnight, all paid for in advance, yet her visa was not granted until six hours before she flew and then she had to return to our organisation's immigration department in order to obtain permission to travel. This last-minute granting of privileges is not uncommon.

We fly to Dubai for a long weekend: what a contrast to our adopted home! We live in an Arab world where the rhythm of the day is set by the call to prayer, where the hot desert wind blows and the ghutra and shayla protecting the wearers' faces offers an obvious solution to the onslaught of the elements (even if it seems a little extreme in the shopping malls). Dubai, on the other hand, is a futuristic cosmopolitan city, with six-lane motorways, a monorail coursing through the city and skyscrapers so tall that as the plane flies up away from the city we remain looking up at the buildings for a long time. The Renaissance towers of St Gimignano come to mind as we look at the bright lights of these modern-day towers. I cannot but smile at the mischievous thought that men's willy-waving spans the centuries.

Staying in the same hotel as we had done ten years ago, we are again enchanted by the manicured lawns, exotic fountains and exquisitely lit inner courtyards serving cocktails and shisha pipes. Admittedly the palm trees encrusted with fairy lights owe more to local taste than ours but still, it is very beautiful. Last time, we were on the edge of town and looked out onto the Gulf and the darkness beyond. Not so now.

We are surrounded by tall towers and in the ocean we see the reclaimed islands known as the Palm, where the buildings unfortunately resemble something out of the communist Eastern Bloc. Our hotel is built along the lines of a desert fort, albeit a very luxurious one, and as we are out of season (the temperature is hitting fifty degrees centigrade with high humidity) we take a suite (cheap at this time of year) which is probably bigger than Lionel's old flat in London.

Most people come to Dubai to shop and we are no different, but it is the gold souq rather than the shopping mall that lures us. I don't really intend to buy anything but the Syrian jeweller's persuasive deals involving convoluted discounts mean that we come away with a tidy cache of jewels for me.

The bustle outside the souq is typically Middle Eastern and we hail several taxis (empty with their for-hire lights on) only to be waved away. Meanwhile a dodgy character in a beaten-up car offers us a lift which, after negotiating the price, Lionel accepts. The car is smelly, noisy and we snuggle into the back with one frayed seat belt between us. The sound of the head gasket about to blow is accompanied by insistent beeps, which we realise indicate lack of petrol when our driver rolls into a garage and asks for twenty dirhams worth of fuel.

Meanwhile he clearly hasn't a clue where he is going and is assiduously avoiding the motorway and the toll charges. Somehow we manage to find our hotel, whereupon we are stopped at the gate by the guard who looks at our car and driver very snootily, then sniffs as the window is wound down and he is treated to the ghastly smell emanating from within.

He waves us through after Lionel intercedes, but our driver has a sudden wobbly and insists on dropping us off just shy of the grand entrance. Frankly the hotel probably wouldn't welcome such a car near their portals and we just want to escape, so we pay the man – plus the price of his petrol – and scurry away.

The incongruity of our lavish hotel room, jewellery purchases and our ride home in a scruffy smelly car running out of petrol will be a subject of Lionel being teased forevermore.

Altogether it is a good break, although there is a stark difference between our adopted home and Dubai. On Fridays in Doha we are treated to the whole service from the nearby mosque whereas here it is the gin palaces and jet skis that destroy the peace with their incessant buzzing and blaring music. I am also intrigued when our Syrian jeweller tells me that, "Your sheikh is prolonging the war by supporting the terrorists and trying to make us all Muslim." Like the rest of the western world I am convinced that Assad and his cronies are the bad guys, but this reminds me that there are normal people caught in the middle of this horrible civil war, who fear for their lives and culture. Presumably our jeweller is one of the Alawite or Christian minorities, but we didn't prolong the conversation.

It never ceases to amaze or shock me how some people here have to endure daily tribulations. I have a Palestinian colleague whose family live on the Gaza strip. He studied in Tel Aviv but was not allowed proper graduation documents because he is an Arab. Not for the first time, I realise what a tolerant, diverse society we come from.

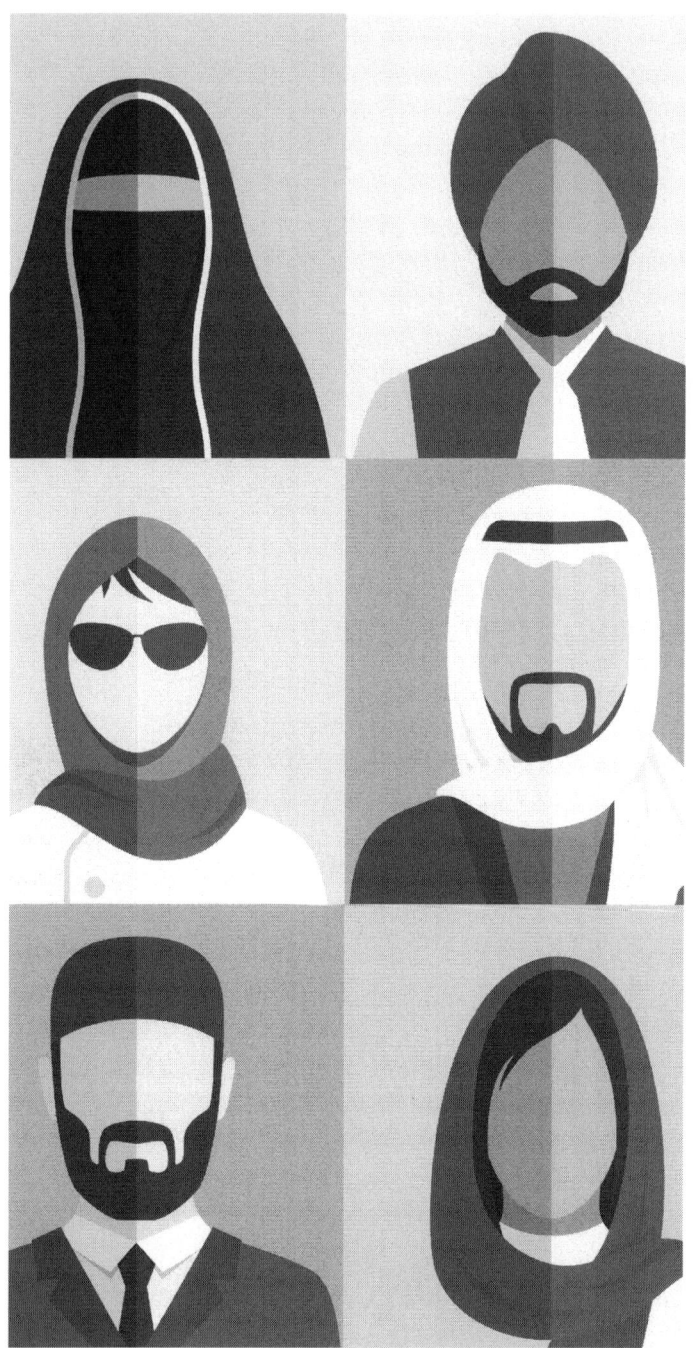

15

A MEDIEVAL FIEFDOM

Agnes, our maid, is a diminutive four foot six inches tall and weighs less than seven stone. Her skin is poor with frequent eruptions of acne, but she has a lovely open smile and lustrous long black hair. She works hard, cleaning thoroughly, pulling out sofas, chairs and even the cooker, so that the whole house is spotless. Her iPhone is plugged into her ears and she sings as she works. Her voice is beautiful and she belts out pop songs with a gusto that belies her size.

At Christmas, she and her fellow maids went out carolling and Agnes sang the solos. She confessed that Christmas is a sad time for her as her two children are in the Philippines and she only travels home once every two years. All her money goes back to her family there. She occasionally asks for medical advice and the latest was how to stop snoring. Apparently one of her room-mates snores loudly and on further enquiry, we discover that she shares a room with five other women.

We know little about this accommodation except that they are expected to be back by 10pm and there was trouble at Christmas when some of the girls stayed out late partying. Memos were delivered to the miscreants. We don't know exactly what this means but to Agnes, it is a serious threat. The ultimate sanction for all ex-pat workers is to be sent home, but we think they all survived.

She would love to live and work solely for us. Our plans are different and when we converted the servants' quarters into a gym, she was convinced that the new furniture was a bed for a new maid. Her delight when she discovered that it was a treadmill being delivered was palpable.

We ask her to stay late one evening in order to help with a supper party and we insist that she eats before we do. I cook a piece of fillet steak for her, which I serve with chips and salad and take to her while she perches on a stool watching television in the gym. When I then serve her some pudding she is quite overwhelmed that anyone would personally serve her and with such delicious food. We leave her happily watching musicals on the TV while we eat with our guests and when I go to ask for her help in between courses, I find her curled up on a couple of cushions, fast asleep. I haven't the heart to wake her.

She is fiercely loyal and refers to "my madame and my sir". Lionel threw out some of his hand-made Italian shirts because the cuffs were frayed and she retrieved them from the waste bin in the bedroom and proudly gave them to the driver who ferries all the maids to and from work. He was delighted, although we are not sure whether he has the cufflinks to go with the double cuffs.

The disparity in incomes is huge and she earns a pittance compared to us, yet still we pay significantly more to her company than many maids earn. Lionel slips her tips every so often and she seems very happy. She is certainly scrupulously honest and if we want her to work overtime she tries to insist that we don't pay extra.

Along with her sunny nature she is extremely scatty. When we were away for a week we asked her to clean and to water the plants. Two days into our holiday, we had a phone call one evening, while settling down to a quiet dinner, to be told that there was water flooding out of our front gate. Because the property is surrounded by twelve-foot-high walls, no one could tell whether the water was emanating from the house or from the garden tap.

We phoned Agnes who went round in a taxi to find everything was fine. We subsequently discovered that one of next door's staff had shimmied over the wall and switched off the tap which Agnes had left open causing the hose to burst and flood the garden ... except most of the plants are in pots and she had failed to water the two newest specimens. Luckily with some judicious drenching on our return, they survived. So Agnes managed to cause a flood while simultaneously dehydrating the plants, but it is difficult to stay cross with her for long. She just giggles while apologising.

She is resourceful too. When, in typical scatty fashion, she took the rubbish out and the door slammed behind her leaving her stranded outside in the road, she borrowed a ladder from next door, climbed onto the wall, straddled it, pulled the ladder over and climbed down our side.

One day she will go home to stay but like so many ex-pat workers, the money here is better and she has to support her family. We berate ourselves in the west for losing our family values, yet in many parts of the world, children are brought up by grandparents and the extended family so that parents earn the money to support them while living thousands of miles away from their young children.

The medical administrator, Dr Mahmod, is an Iraqi who left his home country after the fall of Saddam Hussein. Like many of his compatriots, he welcomed the fall of the dictator, but life in Baghdad became untenable in the aftermath. Bombings and kidnappings became commonplace. He has been here nearly ten years and runs the medical staffing office, which means that he knows everyone, knows how much they are paid, whether they have had complaints against them and of course he converses in Arabic. But as I later discover, all is not quite as it seems.

There is a constant stream of people popping into his office, sharing a pot of Arabic coffee or strong black sweet tea and enjoying a good gossip. He may not be a local but he certainly seems to have *wasta*. He is a large man with an expansive waistline, a droopy moustache and a lugubrious affect. Everything is gloomy in his world until he gets chatting, then he laughs. He is teased by one of the surgeons, who says that there are always bombs in Baghdad when Mahmod has been there to see his father and he must be a secret terrorist. This outrageous comment is treated with a smile and a shrug. It is a bit of black humour and no offence is taken.

Meanwhile he tells me that Qatar has been good to him. He was welcomed, given a job and has been able to educate his girls who are both now at university in Canada. He and his wife have a good life and he can travel freely back to Iraq to visit his aging father.

There are Palestinians here who have no passports, Libyans who are now contemplating going home after many years, Syrians who can no longer go home ... and all these ex-pats, unlike us, are endlessly peripatetic. The ex-pat doctors are well paid but have no pensions and for them there is no stability.

An episode that occurred after about eighteen months into the job brought this into sharp relief. A senior Lebanese consultant, Dr Hanadi, highly respected in the organisation with roles in research and management besides her clinical duties, was summarily suspended. There were allegations that her training in France was bogus and that she did not have the post-graduate qualifications that she claimed. There was a move to simply sack her and put her on a plane, but Dr Mahmod and the team insisted on an investigation. He made phone calls to various institutions in Paris, following which she was completely exonerated and returned to work.

She popped into my office, considerably shaken and wondering how this had happened. The Arabic speakers knew: there had been a whispering campaign instigated by a malicious member of her team. The gossip on Twitter was rife but we Brits heard nothing of this. We think that we are doing well, getting into the culture, but there are always undercurrents of which we have no notion.

Much later she dropped by again.

"I will miss you, Dr Penelope," she said.

"Why? I'm not going anywhere."

"But I am," she responded. "My husband has work here and the lifestyle is good, but I've had enough. The children and I are going back to Paris."

With her western dress and haircut, yet also perfect Arabic, she was a good link between East and West. I was sad to see her go.

On this same note of unexpected outcomes Lionel recently met with the local head of forensic medicine to discuss the lack of post mortem examinations. As one does in this society, initial discussion took them to their past medical lives and it transpired that the forensic physician had been a two-star general in the Iraqi Armed Forces heading their medical services while Lionel was the equivalent two-star in the British military heading medical operations for the opposing side. They are now good friends with many similar values. However, the Iraqi general cannot return home, having been a member of Saddam's army; the British Admiral retains so much more inherent freedom – such meetings teach us so much about the privileges that our society enjoys.

Among these privileges are job security and fair treatment if allegations are made. Not so for poor Mahmod. He appears to have enormous *wasta*, knowing everyone, sharing a joke in Arabic and with fingers in many pies, yet what happens? He is sacked.

His title is Assistant Medical Director, which sounds very grand although his post is middle grade, far junior to me and junior to the consultants, though many hold him in awe. He runs the Medical Staff Office, which - it transpires - is responsible for just about everything including recruitment, annual appraisal, privileges for doctors undertaking operations, compensation, and reward. My role is to look after the professional development of medical staff, so that tallies nicely with the Medical Staff Office and I agree that I will take on Dr Mahmod and his team as part of my responsibilities. Mahmod declares himself very happy with this proposal.

Unfortunately nothing happens. Indecision rules and people are worried that a diminutive female westerner might not be able to manage him. In the event it becomes apparent that no one is managing him (so I couldn't have done worse). Because there are no checks and balances, he does more than he should, making mistakes and ultimately condemning himself by a gross error of judgement. It is a salutary tale of a man promoted beyond his talents and allowed free rein to do things beyond the limits of his competence.

So what happened? I was away in Singapore on an official mission and return to work on a Sunday to be told that Dr Mahmod has been sacked. He received the letter on the Saturday and is never seen again. His office is a shambles and there are personal papers scattered over his desk. There seems to be no process for looking after this man who is now potentially a refugee with no home, no job and no income.

After his departure someone mentions to me, "Pity about Dr Mahmod – he was always good for a prescription," even though Mahmod hadn't practised medicine for over 10 years.

I never discover what happened officially but I subsequently hear from another Iraqi that he has been allowed to stay in his house for a while and someone has taken his possessions home for him. What was his crime? He gave his wife a job. She wasn't exactly working for him and the issue is probably that he facilitated her employment. We will never know the truth but my impression is that his real crime was working in an Arab way in an Arab world that wants to be western and progressive, even though the reality is nearer to a medieval fiefdom.

As I fly in from Singapore I reflect on the insights gained from visiting two academic, high-achieving organisations. I have been discussing strategy and concocting bold plans and now in addition to my main role I am being asked to take over the running of an administrative department where chaos rules. In my former life in the NHS, I have been in charge of such departments, where my role was leadership, team building and strategy, alongside my clinical work. Other, highly competent, admin people ran the day-to-day business. I discover very quickly that such people do not exist with my new responsibility. There are rules but no one follows them or knows them … but then they change all the time.

Maybe the rule is – there are no rules, yet I suddenly become the conduit for the rules and their interpretation. There are processes (probably) but no one knows them or rather they leak out piecemeal and everything is clothed in secrecy. Salaries are very variable even for people doing the same job and this causes immense unrest. Consequently individuals are always asking for salary revisions. I knew this and had been working with Dr Mahmod and others to simplify things and to be fair to him, he had been delighted as he'd been floundering. Only after he left did I fully realise the extent of the problem.

There is a backlog of salary review requests.

"What are we doing about it?" I ask Priyanka, the very beautiful but dippy Indian admin assistant.

"We tell them it is on hold until the next compensation committee meeting," she says, smiling.

This sounds reasonable except that I have never heard of this committee.

"When is the next meeting planned?" I enquire.

"Oh, we don't have one planned."

"Do we have a committee?"

"Well not exactly, well no."

"And how many requests are waiting?"

"Only about three hundred." She beams.

So in a society where money is a huge motivator, we have systematically been lying to senior doctors, who as a result are making waves at high levels and suddenly I am being summoned to sort it out.

The 'learned helplessness' among the staff is endemic. They tell me they need an electronic filing system but they are incapable of articulating their needs; they want me to instruct them but they have no common processes; filing cabinets bulge with incomplete personal files and walking between desks is like stepping through a minefield with piles of files haphazardly distributed over the floor. Uneven piles of papers clutter every available space on every desk. I am notoriously untidy but even I am disquieted. I suggest putting some files away and this is greeted by gasps of horror and explanations about how each pile is crucial to some aspect of the work.

As a consequence of all this disarray, we are constantly bombarded with requests for information on the progress of various functions, such as the recruitment of a senior doctors. Dr Mahmod's office was opposite mine and there was a constant stream of people visiting him. He was affable and there was plenty of laughter, but did they go away appeased? I am not sure. He worked like a vizier in the old Turkish Ottoman court.

All his immense organisational knowledge was in his head, but nothing was written down. His staff were incredibly loyal and as a consequence any rules or policies were kept secret. All the consultants in the organisation, though technically senior to him, were graced only with minimal snippets of information.

Hence they are amazed when I send them electronic copies of the promotion guidelines, as they were never allowed to know these except on a case-by-case basis. This is not unusual. We are currently undergoing what might be loosely described as a redundancy process: in truth, a mass sacking of loyal staff. When we asked the Human Resources department to produce a list of frequently asked questions with typical answers, this is refused.

Dr Mahmod was a product of his culture. He worked on the principle that knowledge is power and he became powerful beyond his limits. He thought that he could ingratiate himself by acquiescing to certain people's demands, but when things went wrong no one could save him. Our western values of transparency, anti-corruption, consistency and fairness have never seemed so important to me as they do now.

It's been a few weeks after the Singapore visit. I am beavering away with the door closed. The Arab way is to keep the door open, so people wander in, disrupting meetings and inappropriately listening to private conversations. Usually I keep to the Arab custom but there is a lot to do on salaries and promotions, trying to extricate us all from the mess left by Mahmod.

Suddenly the door opens and there is the MD smiling at me.

"I was just passing, Penny," she smiled. "How are things?"

I am flabbergasted. She has never dropped by before. I gawp at her.

"The MSO needed a shake-up," she says. "I'm pleased you've taken it on. And by the way, any more thoughts about the Singapore trip?"

We had a good chat and after she leaves I wander into a colleague's office where I am late for an informal meeting. He knows exactly why, as do the rest of the corridor. They are buzzing with the news of the MD coming to see Dr Penelope. My street cred has become stratospheric.

It is all very flattering. I seem to have broken through some invisible ceiling. In spite of the apparent brush-off early on, I am being noticed and appreciated.

The surgeon is tall and sweeps along the hospital corridors majestically, flicking his ghutra over his shoulders and twisting it back over his head. He sports an unshaven look with an almost beard, which is common in these parts. He is affable, diplomatic and once you get to know him, a wonderfully indiscreet gossip. Time management is not a skill that he possesses. The first time I met him, I was kept waiting in his secretary's poky little office for twenty minutes. I was starting to feel irritated when he appeared and hustled me into his office where I was given Arabic coffee and made to feel like the only person in the world who mattered. Our meeting overran and subsequently colleagues told me that being kept waiting for only twenty minutes by Dr Mustafa, was an amazing privilege.

He was chatting in my office with me one day with Dr Mahmod.

"Dr Mahmod," he said, "do you remember that surgeon who worked here, a few years back?"

"No, what was his name?"

"I don't remember. He was a good friend and a nice guy but useless. We had to sack him."

"No, sorry," says Mahmod. "Don't know who you mean."

"Yes you do. What was his name? Got it – Mohammed."

"Ah Mohammed, of course. Lovely man – useless surgeon. We had to sack him."

And this conversation in the context of every other male person being called Mohammed.

Dr Mustafa was educated in the UK and Ireland like many of his medical compatriots and his English, though accented, is fluent and engaging. He chats about his fellow countrymen with a disarming candour. Discussing a tricky senior nurse, he explains that she has a good heart really and anyway, she is a product of the system ... so who can blame some of her dodgy decisions? Then he adds: "She is totally corrupt of course."

He is referring to trips abroad for the purposes of recruiting new staff. Anyone sent on an Official Mission flies first class and receives a hefty daily allowance for their pains, plus an extra four days leave for travel purposes. Is this corrupt? Not really, since it is the rules. There are plenty of sanctimonious Brits who berate the locals for travelling abroad for medical treatment, or for accompanying their families for such treatment, yet the number of Official Missions undertaken by Dr Mustafa and British colleagues is legion. I knew I had made it in the system when I was eventually invited to go on one.

The Singapore trip was my first official mission and I was determined to enjoy my brief time there. We worked hard, visiting hospitals and meeting senior academics. Off stage I stayed in the glorious ex-colonial Raffles Hotel, where I enjoyed an original Singapore Sling cocktail. It was delicious and slipped down a treat, but one was enough if I was ever to stand up unaided. Dr Mustafa was also on the mission but like the other Arabs, was staying in a different unspecified hotel. Probably just as well. They would never have coped with the Singapore Slings.

There are many inconsistencies and anomalies in the system, which Dr Mustafa tries to explain. The problem is that just when you think you understand, something happens and you realise that so much culture is ingrained – as a westerner, you will never really grasp it all.

A typical episode which would never happen in the UK springs to mind. One of the extremely affable senior Arabs was passing my office yesterday. He waved a greeting then wandered in for a chat. He happened to be holding a piece of paper which was a report on a CT scan, which he wondered if I could interpret for him. The patient was the wife of a friend, the referring clinician was not from the appropriate specialty and I then realised that patient confidentiality has a completely different meaning out here. Dr Yousuf, who referred the patient, was probably just using his influence to get a head scan on a friend's wife with headaches.

At home I would have asked judicious questions, but out here it seemed better simply to co-operate and then carry on chatting about growing lemons and mangoes. I have no doubt that the casual walk past my office was deliberate. Did we behave in a similar way years ago? Yes, probably. We certainly looked after each other as junior doctors and prescribing for ourselves and others was common when I was a houseman. These days the General Medical Council takes a dim view of such matters. Back in the UK I had to intervene when a good but naïve young doctor prescribed some antibiotics for a colleague, albeit quite appropriately.

Out here, Lionel was astonished to be regaled with a tale from the previous nightshift. A junior doctor on duty in his Emergency Department had an attack of renal colic, which is intensely acutely debilitating and described in textbooks as exquisitely painful. Certainly a sufferer would be unable to work. So, helpfully, a fellow junior gave the sufferer an injection of morphine and looked after his work for an hour or so, while the drug took effect, before the sufferer returned to his patients.

Apart from the unauthorised use of opiates, goodness knows how the patients fared under the care of a spaced-out doctor with renal colic and opiates surging through his bloodstream. Luckily no one came to harm, but the fact that such an event was even contemplated, let alone executed, shows the huge gap in culture between here and home.

Mustafa works hard and thinks little of seeing patients at any time of the day or night. Scheduling work is a concept of which he has no notion. Operating lists routinely overrun and like many Arabs, he will work late into the evening before going to parties then going to bed long after midnight, only to be awoken by the call to prayer at 4.30am. We westerners wimp out long before that, but then we are bad at taking siestas – unlike the locals who often sleep in the afternoon.

There are examples of excellent medical care here, but even the enlightened ones have difficulty managing their diaries, partly because they don't understand the idea of a diary and partly because plans change at short notice and urgent invitations appear which cannot be refused. I am often asked to meet visiting foreign dignitaries at twenty-four hours' notice, yet I know that visitors from the United States, for example, will have planned their trip weeks in advance.

Relationships and trust are very important. I realise that I am trusted by Dr Mustafa when he is giving a fellow (junior) consultant surgeon some wise advice about how to deal with colleagues (in other words, a bollocking). I discreetly try to leave the room, but he makes me stay.

"She's a good friend and she knows what I mean," he says.

In the end the three of us drank some more coffee and all was well. I would never have imagined myself in such a situation –a Western woman sharing a joke with two traditionally dressed Arabs in a dark office (they are all decorated like the inside of Bedouin tents) while my other western colleagues are made to wait outside in the poky office of the secretary.

My admin assistant Aliya sashays along the corridor with killer heels peeping from below her long black abaya.

Her hair is piled high underneath the long black veil which gives her a regal look and her eyes sparkle and flash with their heavily kohl-painted lids and carefully made-up lashes and eyebrows. We don't see her face but her personality shines forth through her gestures, voice and expressive eyes. Her generosity is legendary and most days she brings in delicious home-made almond flavoured cakes or spicy samosas, which are distributed to all the offices along the corridor by the office boys.

She does no real work but literally pushes bits of paper around her desk and wanders around chatting to her friends and colleagues. Since she is local, her job is guaranteed and she argues that she does more than most, since she is always in on time and tends to stay till the end of the day. She speaks very little English but is very warm to me, hugging me with a warm embrace and calling me her *habibi* while she compliments me on my clothes. The other day she came into my office and closed the door whereupon she whisked away the veil to reveal a heavily made-up but pretty face. She is in her mid-thirties and obviously keen on fashion. Her gleaming smile was spoiled by a lesion on one of her upper teeth. I was starting to commiserate with her when I realised that this was not incipient caries but a diamond that had been encrusted onto the tooth itself and of which she was inordinately proud.

She then raised her abaya to reveal tight leggings and figure-hugging T-shirt. Conversation is limited but she explained that she would dress like this outside of the country but here, the culture is clear. In her tribe she covers her face and seems perfectly content. Another colleague, highly educated, with her postgraduate education completed in London, also covers her face, but lifts her veil when I am in the room alone with her.

Aliya, who does no real work, earns a reasonable

salary and extra benefits simply because she has a job. She and her husband drive large four-wheel-drive cars and were probably given land on which to build a house. There is no Arab Spring here. The Emir is generous with his people but the downside is the lack of motivation. Since the locals don't really need to work, they lack drive and ambition yet in my organisation, the rules are skewed so that locals earn more than ex-pats and only locals can be promoted.

This ridiculous ruling causes tension and friction, particularly in admin and clerical grades where it is rigidly observed. Doctors fare better with promotion opportunities and their salaries are good (but with higher rates of pay for locals) – there are no pensions for ex-pats, whereas when locals decide to retire, they just stop coming to work and carry on being paid as before.

Meanwhile Aliya openly flirts with everyone, flashes her eyes and as she leaves on a Thursday afternoon, briefly lifts her veil and blows me a kiss, while wishing me a good weekend.

Lionel is particularly discomforted by the obvious flirting. One particular junior member of his staff is very blatant. We call her Fatima the Flirt – she openly describes how she feels about him, asks him about his wife and if I am out here and mentions that she herself is unmarried. She then flutters her eyelashes at him and proceeds to lift her skirts while asking him to examine her knee.

"You're a doctor – will you look at my swollen knee?"

He has never even seen her face.

16

BAD NEWS AND GOOD MEN

I t is Ramadan again. The shops are full of special offers and Ramadan tents have sprung up everywhere.

Fasting and feasting is the order of the day. They all put on weight and laugh at me when I tell them that I lost weight last year because I was fasting. It has a certain logic to me but that's because I go home, have a normal supper after the six-thirty call to prayer and am in bed by half past nine, whereas they leave work at about one in the afternoon, have a sleep then are ready to get up and party through the night, plus a fair amount of praying of course.

Work diminishes as no one is there for half the day. It is tricky for those operating or working in the Emergency Department, especially as they can't even drink water: in temperatures reaching fifty degrees Celsius and more, this is frankly unsafe.

One of my duties is to chair a committee that is overseeing the staffing of a new hospital. The opening of this hospital is delayed and we don't know when there will be any patients, but in the meantime interviews take place in order to choose suitable candidates to work in this gleaming new institution. The rules have been clearly stated, namely that only doctors with western qualifications will be accepted and those with Arab boards will not. I suppose it should be flattering that our degrees are considered so prestigious, but it still seems harsh. The Arab boards are no pushover and often achieved against many odds.

The venue for the examinations moves between different Arab countries and this means that sometimes a candidate is ineligible to sit for the exam simply because he cannot obtain a visa for that country. Since they are held infrequently, this can seriously hamper someone's career. I am told by several sources that sometimes candidates are barred from sitting the exams by the organisation. This is the case for foreign nationals such as Palestinians who are living here, often without passports, because until recently they were deemed to be stateless.

One resourceful Palestinian did his post-graduate training in Israel and has excellent references from there, but was unable to gain the full certificate because non-Israelis were barred from doing the final exams. It is staggering how many of our staff have either lived through, or are escaping from, areas of conflict. Syrians, Libyans, Lebanese and Iraqis are commonplace. They are survivors and life for them continues to be tenuous.

The interview results are ready but suddenly everyone is stalling. "We don't know when the hospital will open so let's keep quiet for the moment" is the message.

I am appalled, arguing that these people's livelihoods are at stake and they should know where they stand, whether the news is good or bad. It should be added that those without posts in the new place are at serious risk of losing their jobs altogether since services are transferring *en masse.* However the managing director has promised to keep such people in employment here for two years, so they will have time to seek new work elsewhere and we might be able to keep some of them in managerial and administrative roles. Still the Arabs are stalling.

They are worried about the press. They are worried that rejected applicants might leave before the transfer of services (and why should they not?) but mainly it appears they don't want to give bad news and they will do anything to defer a decision. We see this with patients too.

Doctors here are happy to talk to relatives, but balk at telling the patient herself that she has breast cancer. Conversations in committee rooms proceed in circuitous fashion with decisions carefully not being made. There is always someone higher up who can, or must, be consulted so decisions are deferred pending the minister's opinion, for example. In this case, I pushed back hard and managed to persuade the committee that we must inform candidates of the results of the interviews.

Support comes from an unexpected source, namely a highly religious, dedicated senior doctor who agreed that the uncertainty and tensions among his staff are helping no one, least of all the patients. This particular doctor, Dr Hassan, is a small man with a long grey beard, flowing robes and twinkling eyes. He could be a benevolent gnome, but if encountered at Heathrow airport I suspect that he would not pass through security services easily. He is undoubtedly a good man, although I still find it disconcerting that he won't shake my hand.

Dr Hassan and I are working together to review certain services. The genetics service is a case in point: diseases which result from the high degree of intermarriage are seldom seen in the west. The rate of consanguineous marriage is said to be of the order of seventy percent and is defined by marriage between second cousins or closer. In reality, first cousins often marry and stay within the tribe, so the gene pool becomes even more concentrated. He shows me a family tree where first cousins were married whose own parents were also first cousins in the same family. Tragically, of the five offspring of this latest marriage, four had serious rare genetic conditions. Dr Hassan and I discuss the issues with the consultant geneticist. It is now possible to screen *in utero* and I wonder if termination is allowed in Sharia law.

I hesitate to ask the question in case of giving offence, but the conversation is frank and humanitarian. Such terminations before a certain stage of pregnancy are permitted and encouraged and counselling is offered. Much research is being done and new conditions are being discovered along with the causative genes.

We discuss the coming holidays and Dr Hassan tells me that he is going to Mecca on a mini-pilgrimage, an *Umrah* (lesser pilgrimage). This is unlike the *Hajj*, which must be performed once in every Muslim's life and takes place in a particular lunar month.

I know all this because Dr Hassan kindly gave me a leaflet on Islam, written especially for non-Muslims. What is fascinating is how so many of the tenets of this religion are similar to Christianity, although the conclusion that the Bible predicts the coming of the Prophet Mohammed through the gospel of St John is probably stretching a point. Daily life for Muslims in this part of the world revolves around their religion, which also imposes standards of behaviour in daily living and recognises the importance of family and kinfolk. The sadness is that the fundamentalists have subverted it and we have threats of terrorism from extremists who bear no resemblance to the normal people living their lives in the Middle East.

17

THE DARK SIDE

A consultant colleague came into my office last Thursday afternoon in order to ask for my help. He is an Arab but a non-Qatari. I had never met him before and he exuded a curious mix of agitation and resignation. He thrust a letter into my hand which was written by someone in the corporation, dismissing him from his post.

It was unambiguous but there was no explanation. I was shocked and asked him if he had received any warning.

"Nothing," he said. "I am on a three year contract; I've done about twenty months."

It occurred to me that perhaps he was failing in his clinical duties but he reassured me.

"No, my work is good. Ask anyone. Anyway, I will be OK. I've been offered a job back in the UK but I don't want to disrupt my children's schooling too much. They might let me stay till the end of the school term."

"But," I said, "this is appalling, frankly unbelievable.

There must be some reason for your dismissal."

I rang his boss who assured me that this was an excellent doctor, in a shortage specialty and he didn't want to lose him.

"Well, perhaps my wife failed the CID scrutiny," he said. "We used to work here in the past and she left to finish her training in England. Maybe that upset someone."

I spoke to the Qatari Medical Director of his hospital who was more expansive.

"It is political and we will never know why," said the director. "The decision will have come from the Ministry of the Interior and there is no point in trying to speak to them as they are all shits".

This comment from a local.

I spoke to someone in Human Resources who said that in such cases they often could extend the notice period for the sake of the children's schooling. Ten minutes later she rang back and said there was nothing they could do. I subsequently discovered that five senior doctors were being expelled from the country for no reason, except that they are all Shia Muslims from Iraq and the predominant group here are Sunni. We joke about being 'put on a plane' but it really does happen.

We rail against stringent health and safety rules in the west, but here such issues are a mere detail. Lionel is pleased to discover that his hospital had a valid Fire Certificate, just a pity that the emergency exits are locked and no one knows the evacuation procedures. He is reassured that he has nothing to worry about because there is an in-date certificate. Maybe that was the same reassurance given to the (British) Executive Director in charge of stores before he was thrown into jail.

His incarceration was despite the fact that he had complained to higher authorities about his organisation's fire safety, but his pleas had been ignored. Regardless of his propriety, he was now being held personally responsible for the fire.

The fire was in a medical stores warehouse on a Thursday and someone had to be blamed. So the Director was arrested and imprisoned at a weekend with no recourse to lawyers, diplomatic aid or even a visit from the executive team in the corporation. He spent several days in prison before being released on bail.

The supply chain into the country is poor at the best of times and there is a certain degree of stockpiling. Unfortunately the stocks were cinders and we had to cancel theatre sessions and fly urgent medical items in from neighbouring Arab states, who currently are not always sympathetic to our plight. A recent pan-Arab international conference was boycotted by local GCC (Gulf Cooperation Council) countries as they are dismayed at our Qatari government's stance on the Egyptian question. The Arab Spring in Egypt resulted in the overthrow of President Hosni Mubarak and brought the Muslim Brotherhood and the Islamist president Mohamed Morsi to power. Qatar supported Morsi but the other Gulf States were concerned that this meant Qatar was supporting terrorist movements such as so-called Islamic State. Who knows what is really going on? It is likely to be murky whatever the truth.

An Englishwoman was murdered outside a well-known hotel and her burnt body subsequently discovered in the desert. The perpetrators were caught as they returned to the scene to check their deed and the crime was widely reported in the international press. We do hear of such crimes going unreported and our colleagues in the Emergency Department see bodies brought in, but there is no investigation into the cause of death.

Back in the hospital a particular felony was almost

certainly averted by the swift action of the CEO and medical director of one of the hospitals. The story is that a male nurse was found stroking the arm of a young female patient. The family discovered and were incensed; quite rightly so. Murder would seem to be an over-the-top response but the Qatari Medical Director, a deeply religious man, was convinced that if we didn't get the hapless nurse out of the country, he would be whisked off into the desert, retribution would ensue and he would not live to tell the tale. The hospital smuggled him to the airport and managed to get him on a plane before the brothers turned up in a posse of Land Cruisers.

Throughout our time in Qatar, we constantly ask ourselves, "Can we live in this society?"

What is our problem? We like our Arab colleagues (in the main), we are well paid and we are constantly fascinated by this different society – but sometimes its values are so very different from ours that we feel morally compromised. There are times when we feel unable to do our jobs properly. Other ex-pats are more pragmatic, "Keep your head down, Lionel," is one piece of advice. "Don't rock the boat."

My husband isn't very good at keeping a low profile, particularly when he believes he is in the right. An example is the plan to decentralise the finance department. In theory this is an excellent idea. Each hospital in the country would have control over its own budget, hence using resources more wisely. Plans for this process are racing ahead but it isn't going smoothly. No one likes change and the power of passive resistance should never be underestimated.

Lionel is in a top-level meeting where the managing director asks whether financial decentralisation is going well.

"Yes," comes the group reply. "All the hospitals now

have complete responsibility for their budgets."

"Good," she says, "because the Minister is uncomfortable with this decentralisation."

Lionel, of course, speaks up. "He would be even more uncomfortable if he knew that finance had been devolved but without any financiers to advise within the hospitals."
She glares at him down the table. He is obviously trouble. The others are glibly telling her what she wants to hear: Lionel is telling the truth. And his staff support him. At another meeting with the minister and the MD, he makes the same mistake of saying how it is. Later she reprimands him.

"I do apologise," he says. "I am completely loyal to you. If you'd briefed me on your constraint then I would have kept quiet."

The problem is a disconnection between the grandiose plans of the government and the reality on the ground. Beautiful new hospitals are being built but never finished, so the work goes on in underequipped shabby wards in old buildings. A world-ranking Academic Health System to rival Harvard or Cambridge is planned. Professors from around the world are recruited with promises of wonderful laboratories for blue skies research. They soon find their way to my office with their tales of woe. "But there is no lab," or "There are no research staff," or "Everyone is so busy that they have no time to even consider research" are comments I hear repeatedly.

There are some excellent doctors and nurses struggling to treat patients in an infrastructure more akin to the 1970s than the twenty-first century. In my working life in the NHS at home, I have witnessed and effected huge changes, over thirty years. In Qatar we are trying to do that in three years, in a society that is only just emerging from living as nomads in the desert.

There is an element of *emperor's new clothes*. The courtiers happily applaud the superficial froth but there is nothing underneath. Some of the froth is quite good fun, however. The minister pays an unscheduled call to Lionel in his office. Lionel's hospital is brand new, beautiful and well equipped but already too small.

"We need an extension and a more office space," says Lionel.

"You are doing a good job. I hear excellent reports about you and I agree. I will sign off the building plans tomorrow," responds the minister.

Within weeks, work is nearing completion on his new Emergency Department extension and a temporary Portakabin has been erected. But what a Portakabin! The staircases are marble and the office walls are panelled in the finest wood embellished with gold leaf. There is still no budget to raise the wages of the impoverished office workers, however. It is an extraordinary world.

We discuss our future while on annual leave, sailing in the Aegean. It is fascinating to reflect that when we first visited Turkey it was exotic and different. After two or more years in the Middle East, Turkey feels positively European. Drinking a glass of wine at a quayside restaurant while skimpily clad Turkish girls saunter past is very different to our Qatari experiences. The call to prayer still dominates but no one seems to take any notice, unlike Qatar where the mosques are full five times a day.

As our time passes, we are both becoming unsettled. We have achieved much and are well respected by our Arab colleagues, but we sense trouble ahead. Lionel has come to a natural break point in his role. There is a new ministry named the Ministry of Administrative Development, a name straight out of *Yes Minister*. Except these civil servants have an Arab mentality, not a Whitehall one.

Power struggles are in play between the MOAD and the Health ministries. There never has been a proper budget allocation and it is getting worse. Recruitment is nigh impossible: every newcomer to the country has to be vetted by the Ministry of Interior and this process takes months.

The rules are predictably opaque. We are told, unofficially, that certain nationalities will never get in. Sudanese and possibly Egyptians are on the blacklist, yet the country is full of such ex-patriots, well-educated and good workers. Where is the truth? I try to recruit an Englishman of Pakistani descent. His credentials are good and he is desperately needed in my department, but after a year of getting nowhere, I concede that he will never be let in, for whatever reason.

Meanwhile Andrea, my British assistant, has left. Her husband works in Dubai so she was going back to their apartment there every weekend, for which she needed an exit permit, signed by me, for every trip. We tried to circumvent the system by signing a pile in advance but when she was ill and couldn't simply go home, it was all too much. She has resigned. I try to promote Joramae into her position but to no avail.

Understandably, the Qataris are keen to promote their own staff. There is a positive discrimination policy of 'Qatarisation', which means that all jobs should be offered to a Qatari first. *Their country and their rules*, we think, except that jobs are given to Qataris who have no experience of the job in hand and who then never turn up for work.

Non-Qataris are not allowed to be promoted except when a Qatari wishes to break the rules. Then a favoured ex-pat will be promoted internally. Such actions cause covert accusations of foul play and discontent among the other workers.

In many ways, Qatar is an ambitious state with a drive to modernise and improve. There is an awareness that the oil may dry up and something else will need to sustain the country. Dubai has settled for tourism, but Qatar has little natural beauty and its society is much more traditional, hence the suggestion of a knowledge economy as the way forward. So there is an Education City, a Medical City and a Science and Technology Park. Good work undoubtedly ensues but there is also much froth and misplaced energy.

For example, among our doctors we have multiple nationalities with diverse qualifications. Some are extremely good doctors, but have no specialist degrees to prove their credentials. Others are also-rans, who do the basic work to support the consultants. It's an archaic system and not entirely fair as there is definite prejudice against some nationalities.

"We must change and modernise," announces the minister. "If our hospitals are to be world ranking then we can only employ doctors with the best qualifications."

He has a good point but the system cannot change overnight. As usual, passive resistance ensues and nothing happens.

I have some sympathy with the minister's views. He wants the best for his country; the problem is that he doesn't understand how medicine works and no one has the courage to challenge him. They just shout at me instead. Of course I would happily discuss matters with the minister but no one will allow that to happen. I feel frustrated with the system and angry on behalf of the doctors whose lives are about to be unfairly disrupted.

The minister discovers the inaction and put the pressure on our MD. She transmits his fury to my boss.

"Why has nothing happened?" she fumes. "The minister has discovered and he is furious! Sort it or I will

dismiss these doctors who haven't got full qualifications!"
It turns out that poor Dr Mahmod was partly to blame but then he'd had no direction. It falls to me and my new boss to sort out. As I start to delve into the issues I discover the tangled web and it certainly influences my decision that it's time to leave.

Both Lionel and I feel we are being asked to do things that we find very uncomfortable. Hospital beds are much in demand, but Lionel is asked to provide one so that a Sheikha can have her own personal maid sleeping next to her. We signed up to the system but it is becoming clear that the conflict with our own values is too much to bear.
Why am I so bothered? I have always been clear that patients are my first concern and the last thing I would sanction would be poorly qualified doctors giving poor care. Of course it isn't like that: many of these non-Qatari doctors have been in post for years. Highly experienced, they've taught their junior staff who have then been promoted above them. It isn't that they are lazy but they often are not allowed to sit the examinations for the Arab boards.

Sometimes these doctors have unique skills, such as the Iraqi General who was working in the morgue. Post mortems are not forbidden in Muslim societies, but local customs mean they are very infrequently undertaken. So suspicious or unexpected deaths become very difficult to assess. The Iraqi pathologist had much experience and was the only person in the country who could deal with unexpected deaths. Not only the hospital staff but the Ministry of the Interior wondered how they would manage without him.

I like to think that we could have dealt with this problem in a managed way. Further training perhaps? But in Qatar? For foreign nationals? Apparently not. They are to be dismissed. The end result is all that matters, never mind the human fall-out.

But it is not just the humanitarian aspects that concern me and many of my Qatari colleagues. There is a pragmatic element. How will the country appear in the eyes of the world if swathes of doctors are suddenly sacked for no good reason? Many of these doctors are Palestinian, technically refugees. They have no passports, many have lived in the Gulf for decades, have children in school and literally have nowhere else to go. Imagine the diplomatic furore if these people are summarily dismissed and ejected from the country?

We can't appoint doctors and nurses fast enough to cope with demand. The population is increasing exponentially, mainly with construction workers preparing the buildings and infrastructure for the World Cup. Families are also arriving and the pressure on maternity and paediatric services is immense. Yet the government refuses to discuss a reasonable way forward with us in the hospital sector.

I put forward action plans that are rejected, or at least accepted *then* rejected for unfathomable reasons. Qatari consultants lobby me vociferously about individual doctors at risk. "The minister doesn't understand," they say. "You must not let this happen!" I feel powerless.

Nevertheless I look into every case, about hundred and fifty. I meet them all to discuss the realities of their situation. There is a lot of denial, then pleading; grown men in tears in my office, worried for their families.

We try to emphasise the point about Qatar's status on the world stage. Yet no one can reach the MD. She is always away or meetings are cancelled. The chiefs are as powerless as me. Questions are already being asked about the World Cup processes and the football association,

FIFA. We are trying to save face on behalf of the minister, yet inexplicably no one is allowed near him.

It is exasperating and frankly heart-breaking. This is not why I went into medicine and it is certainly not in the interests of the patients. I try to make sense of it all: I can't stop the process but I could limit the damage. If people have to go, then at least make it like a redundancy process, with final salaries and other benefits.

In the end Middle Eastern procrastination allows many people to buy time. Some manage to do their exams and become eligible to stay, some get jobs elsewhere, some retire and some stay in complete denial. Their letters of termination of contract are distributed not long before I leave the corporation.

Building teams and encouraging high morale in such a *milieu* is difficult but not impossible. Rising to the challenge was actually quite fun and we both managed it. Nevertheless, things are not going to improve and our initial enthusiasm is starting to flag. More to the point there are personal things at home that sharpen the mind – the birth of our grandchildren plus a sick mother-in-law – and clinch the decision to return early.

We return to Qatar from our UK annual leave in September of 2014 with a plan to hand in our resignations and be home by Christmas.

This is easier said than done. Lionel goes first. He has completed the job he was given as CEO of the Heart Hospital. The management team are in good shape. Prior to his arrival there was no team, no meetings to discuss policy, simply a collection of disparate Arabs getting things done by the age-old method of *he who shouts loudest achieves the result he wants.* Now, the American-based external regulators, Joint Commission International, inspects the hospital and pronounced it the best-run they have ever assessed in the country. Praise indeed.

But the plan was always to appoint a CEO who was also a Cardiologist. Lionel is a doctor but not that specialty and although the hospital staff (including the Cardiology ex-minister) pleads for him to be kept on, it is to no avail. Face-saving is paramount in this culture.

So Lionel is to be moved. No shame there, but no one will tell him where he is going. So he resigns. And all hell breaks loose.

Mohammed, his deputy, interrupts him one morning.

"Dr Lionel, the MD wants to see you."

"OK, when?"

"Now!" he retorts.

"Fine," says Lionel, "I'll get one of the drivers to take me over to her office in corporate headquarters."

Mohammed looks astonished "But you don't understand," he says. "She is here. She has come specially to see you."

This is unheard of: she never goes to see people on their territory, apart from the ex-minister.

She spends a long time with Lionel, telling him how much she values his work. How she wants him to be her trouble-shooter, how she doesn't want him to leave. But she doesn't offer him a specific job and anyway, the die has been cast.

The knock-on effect, quickly apparent to her and others, is that I will be going too. I dread telling my team. They are now settled in their new offices and I have circumvented a crazy plan to move them again. Meanwhile they have organised a teaching session for all the medical secretaries from the country's hospitals. Suddenly they all have pride in their work and they believe that I am their protector.

There are tears when I tell them I am going but they

rally and decide that at least they can organise a good leaving party. This is a huge secret and I have to be complicit in pretending I know nothing about it.

Because of all the changes I have made to contracts, promotion policy and pay, the senior doctors are distraught. "What can we do to make you change your mind?" they ask. One senior Arab physician puts his head in his hands. "This is a disaster," he says. "You cannot go. What will we do?" To be fair, he is rather given to histrionics and I reassure him that the world will not end if I go home.

It is all very flattering but needs to be put into perspective. Yes, they like me but they are also used to me. They don't want change and worry about who might come next. Still, nice to hear from Dr Mustafa who sighed, "The good people always go."

My own immediate boss is extremely worried about how he will cope without me, although very understanding, so we make an agreement. I will give four months' notice instead of the usual three and he will ensure that I'll be put up in a five-star hotel for the final month when Lionel has already returned to the UK. This latter stipulation is important because of the difficulties of leaving the country: I want no impediment to my easy departure once Lionel has gone.

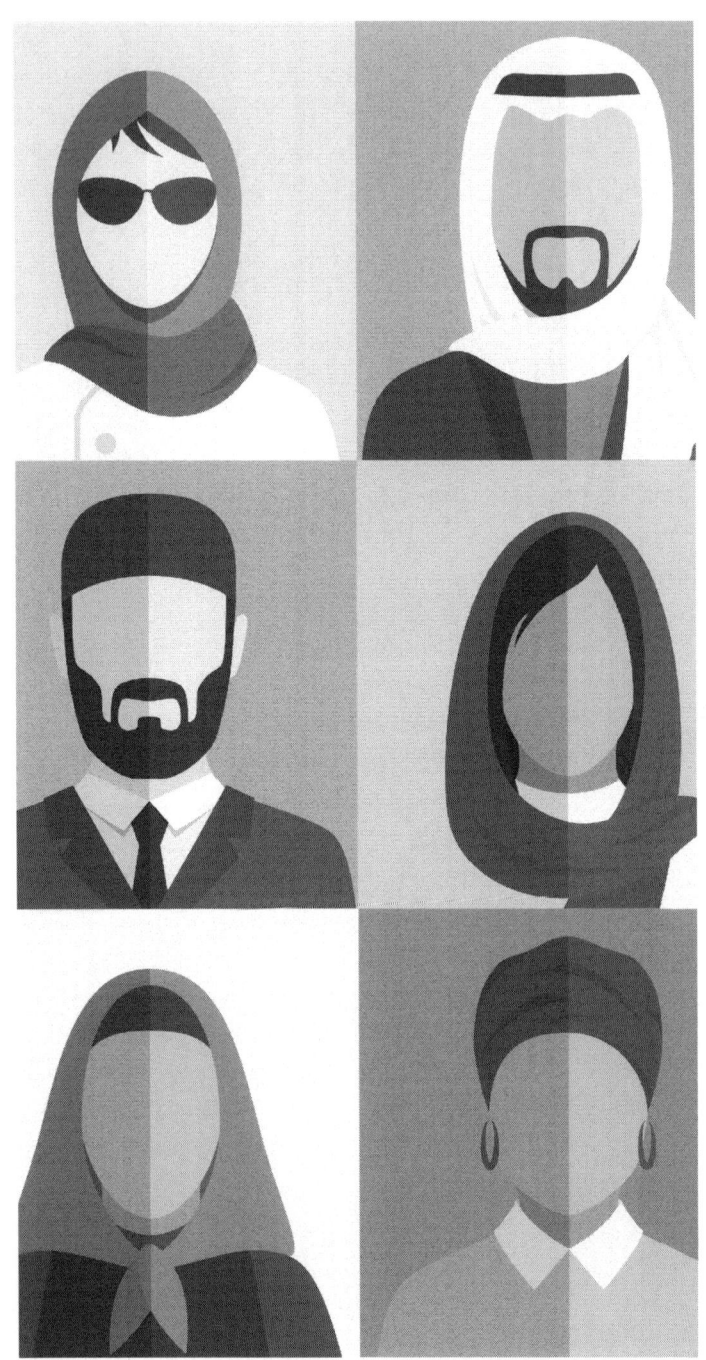

18

FAREWELLS

In spite of the threats of being put on a plane and chucked out of the country at a moment's notice, the reality of leaving at will, as it were, is very different. The country and the corporation are paranoid that leavers might have unpaid debts. This fear stems from the crash of 2008 when the economy collapsed overnight in Dubai. Expats, in their haste, left with the clothes they stood up in. Porsches, Ferraris and other such expensive cars were abandoned, littering the roadside on the way to the airport; tenancy agreements and credit card arrangements were ignored. The wealth had dried up and there was nothing left to stay for.

So there is a long list of procedures to be completed before we can receive our final salary and be allowed to leave the country. True to form, no one knows the rules exactly and certainly no one is going to tell us. Those who have gone before have left few clues. We reckon they were so relieved to be off that compiling a checklist for others was not their priority. So like everyone else, we muddle through.

Leaving the house is the most onerous task. Everything has to be left in pristine condition, even to the extent of taking down curtains and blinds.

"But we have good curtains," we explain to Mr Khalid from Housing. "The new tenants might wish to keep them."

He smiles comfortingly then shakes his head.

"Housing is in short supply. You must know who will take over. Tell us and we will talk to them."

"No, Dr Penelope. Just take everything down. This is all too difficult to arrange."

Our house had been completely unfurnished so we had bought white goods, cooker, fridge and so on.

"Mr Khalid, can we not sell these on to the next person?"

Again, the head shook.

"Or even leave them free of charge?"

No, it would appear this was against all rules and the house must be cleared.

"Including all the plants," he adds.

It is tempting to simply leave everything and pay for any perceived damages, but this is inadvisable. Three inspections are made and if unsatisfactory then final salaries will be docked and the precious exit permit refused. Lionel agrees to sort out the domestic arrangements, leaving me to work and then calmly move into the hotel with him for my final month in post.

Nothing is ever calm in the Middle East. We set about selling all the furniture. Websites abound, with legends such as *Qatar Living*. We advertise an item then wait for the offers to come flooding in. We bargain hard with one man, who gets a good deal on a television. He then turns up in a beaten-up van, gives us a toothless grin and says he has no money. Could he have it for free? He doesn't look like a wealthy man but he is trying to rip us off.

"Give me the money or you don't get the goods," says Lionel sternly.

Suddenly our buyer remembers the cash under the dashboard, but still tries to bargain us down further. We are not playing his game and he gives up, hands over the money and drives off with the TV in the boot and a cheery wave.

We sell a large sideboard to a colleague. He turns up one Saturday morning in a lorry driven by an elderly Arab.

"It's heavy, Dave," I warn, "but the three of you will cope."

"I don't think my man understands that bit of the deal," replies Dave. "He's not shifting from that lorry."

Sure enough, the elderly Arab watched while Lionel, Dave and I struggle to load his truck.

We have some beautiful specimen plants in large tubs. A haughty Syrian lady from along the road buys the lemon tree.

"I'm going out now," she informs us, "You can get your men to bring the tree when I return."

Except we have no men to move trees. I pop in to see my friend Suman from the garden centre. He's always had a soft spot for me and happily complies with my request for a few chaps to come and shift plants, for a small fee.

So at the appointed time we have four men with a large lemon tree in the road in the scorching heat, but no Syrian lady and no reply from the house. I am furious. But Lionel has a plan.

"I'll break in and open the garage door from the inside, then we can dump the lemon tree in her courtyard," he says.

So he shimmies over the wall and our chaps are positioning the tree when she swans in, not having noticed that we are technically trespassing. We pay the garden centre men who leave, then she has the gall to pop round half an hour later.

"I don't like the position of the tree," she announces. "Tell your men to come and move it."

Her husband, by contrast, is delightful. An academic who had trained in France and America, he is the patriarch of the family. His niece has arrived from Syria to live with them, and his adult son also lives at home, but his mother sadly died before she was due to leave his beleaguered homeland. Every day he speaks to relatives there. The situation is worsening and I wonder how his Syrian based extended family will cope. Will they join the trail of refugees crossing Turkey?

We hear that bank accounts need to be closed. This is a worry. How will our salaries be paid? How will we pay our bills? Luckily the rumour is wrong: credit cards are the issue. They have to be relinquished ninety days before we leave the country. Lionel goes first. About three weeks later I follow and give up my card. We check that Lionel is OK as he will be leaving before me.

"Your card has only just been cancelled, sir," advises the bank clerk.

"What!" Lionel exclaims. "But I relinquished it weeks ago."

"Sorry sir, but we have only just cancelled it at the bank. There may be a problem with you leaving the country. It is now less than ninety days."

We are outraged.

"But this is the bank's fault," insists Lionel.

The clerk is unfazed, "Don't worry; we can keep a deposit from your account, in case there are any outstanding debts."

"There are no debts," we say. "Anyway, how much deposit?"

"Fifty thousand riyals," he replies and smiles sweetly.

A mere bagatelle of about ten thousand pounds! This is getting serious and there's no contrition whatsoever from the bank who had cocked up.

The whole thing is a nonsense anyway, as the banks do not allow overdrafts and credit cards are automatically paid off each month. Luckily Lionel never has to find his putative deposit and the first exit hurdle is done.

Utilities, water, electricity, phone and internet all have to be closed down and paid up. Inevitably this is as complicated as it was when we arrived. Timeliness is poorly understood in the Arab world: cancel the electricity too soon and you are cut off the following day, leave it too late and you can't leave the country because they haven't received your final bill.

What to do? Behave like an Arab.

Our Arab colleagues have no notion of the stress we are under. "Just get a boy to do it," they advise. So we do. Ayoub, one of Lionel's hospital's drivers, goes to the utility companies to sign everything off. He whizzes round the hospital, signing off the meaningless checklist. He passes by my office one afternoon beaming and proudly announcing, "Hello ma'am. You know me. I am Dr Lionel's boy!"

My 'boy' is Ibrahim, the Chief Aide on my corridor. I slip him some dosh and he spends many hours and days doing irrelevant tasks such as guaranteeing the return to the laundry of white coats (even though I've never worn one and have never been allocated any).

We have to relinquish our passports. This is uncomfortable and the gilded cage metaphor becomes all too real. I want mine returned as soon as possible so I go personally to the hospital immigration department, accompanied by my henchmen, Ibrahim, who speaks several Indian languages, and Aliya, veiled Qatari lady. I figure this duo will be able to cut through the bureaucracy. It starts well.

We walk into the cramped office, packed with people of all nationalities who part, allowing us to march up to the front. I keep silent but glide in behind them like Lady Bountiful. Can you imagine blatant queue-jumping like that in the UK? I am afraid I have no compunction. This is necessary and expected.

It is to no avail. Lots of Arabic, Urdu, Hindi and a bit of Pidgin English, eyelash fluttering, arm waving and summoning of supervisors … but the answer is an emphatic "No". They will keep my passport as long as necessary, with no explanation whatsoever. We shuffle off, beaten, and I take Aliya for a consolation coffee and cake in the hospital Starbucks.

The house is nearly empty. The curtains have gone, carpets are rolled up ready for shipping home, and the garden is once more a barren wasteland. Ayoub and his mates come over to tidy up the holes in the walls made by picture hooks and the like. A blob of plaster with a covering of paint is all that is needed. We have already advised Ayoub on which shades of paint to buy in small tester pots. Ayoub and the gang fill the holes then proudly demonstrate the painting materials: four pots of paint and one paintbrush. They then proceed to cover one hole and stand back proudly surveying the result.

"This colour is wrong, Dr Lionel," pronounces Ayoub.

"No, it's still wet, so we can't be sure yet," we say.

Ten minutes later no one has moved. The awful truth dawns: we are paying them to watch paint dry.

I take the one paintbrush and test a different area. Ayoub is almost apoplectic.

"No madam, please let me."

They then proceed to systematically paint each hole in order while carefully washing and drying the brush in between. It takes four men and four hours. Luckily they are nice chaps and very inexpensive. We have a pile of stuff that we were unable to sell.

"Take what you want," we say.

They take the lot.

Leaving is a wrench. When I first arrived, I was wary of making eye contact with the Arabs, but my reticence was misplaced. "We like your big smile," they told me, "and Islam tells us you should smile and be friendly." I took their advice and started to freely greet people in the corridors, in the lift.

In the final few weeks, I pass a couple of Paediatricians deeply engrossed in conversation in the main hospital concourse. I know them well and don't wish to appear rude, so as I walk past I say:

"*As-salaam alaikum.*"

"*Wa-alaikum-salaam,*" they reply. Then Dr Mohammed looks up. "Oh it's Dr Penelope. How are you? Is it true you're leaving?"

We chat for a while and they express their regret at my going. They are very polite and would say that. Even so, I reflect on how things had changed from my first few weeks when I was wary of greeting Arabs. Now I am happily conversing in Arabic.

My farewell to the MD is very different to my arrival. This time she makes a point of requesting me to come and say good-bye, which I do.

Interrupting her meeting, she stands up, gives me a big hug and says, "Well Penny, you have certainly made your mark here. We don't want to lose you but we understand."

Family always comes first in the Arab world so the birth of our grandchildren plus a sick mother-in-law is justification for leaving, without loss of face on either side.

Arab generosity is renowned. We receive many leaving gifts, often from unexpected sources. A large bouquet appears in my office one day, from a senior female Arab executive. She is known to be tricky but we have established a reasonably good working relationship. Within the mass of flowers is a small box that I assume contains chocolates. "The aides along the corridor will eat those," I think to myself. "Still I'd better look inside first."

Where I find a beautiful diamond ring. Small diamonds exquisitely crafted in three types of gold; white, yellow and rose. Pearls and gold bracelets for me, cufflinks for Lionel and a total of seven watches between us follow. We are overwhelmed. One of my best offers ever comes after I sold my car and am renting an inferior model, "Take one of the Porsches," invites one of my Qatari team members, who comes from a wealthy family. Tempting, but I politely decline.

These episodes make us realise how truly generous the Arabs are. They have nothing to gain: we are going home yet they give us expensive gifts knowing they might never see us again. We know we will miss our Arab friends and even with the frustrations of the last few months we never wish we'd not embarked on this amazing adventure.

Our leaving parties are pure theatre. We hosted one ourselves before we left the house, which was similar to the *HMS DRAGON* affair. Another balmy evening under the stars and the expat guests are joined by a number of Arab guests who come to enjoy the food and conversation but not the wine.

Not all Arabs are so reticent about alcohol. Dr

Abdulfatir wants to take us out to dinner.

"Where would you like to go?" he asks. "There are some good Arab restaurants down on the corniche, or we could go to the Italian restaurant in the Radisson. It's very good and we can drink wine there," he adds mischievously. I take the hint. "The Italian," I decide.

We meet to find him already ensconced with a pint of beer in front of him. Excellent food and conversation ensue.

"So you don't bring your wife to dinner with you?"

"No." He shakes his head. "She wouldn't come, she's very religious."

"What does she think of you drinking beer?"

"She doesn't know."

"But can't she smell it on your breath?"

"That's no problem," he says, smiling. "I tell her it's the salad dressing."

Lionel's hospital send-off comes first. The lecture theatre in the Heart Hospital is packed. Presents are given and there are photos and eulogies from one staff member after another.

His Head of Security is a burly, thick-set Arab who sports the swarthy unshaven look. One look at him and potential trouble-makers cringe. Security is necessary as Arab families could be difficult when accompanying sick relatives to hospital, especially at night. He has always greeted Lionel with a cheery, "Hello, boss," and the day of the party he arrives in Lionel's office looking completely incongruous with a huge bunch of roses held against his immaculate white thobe.

"For you, boss," he grunts, embracing him with kisses to each cheek. Nestling among the roses is a new smartphone.

My 'do' is similar with the lecture theatre in the

Women's Hospital cordoned off. Again there are presents, eulogies and the whole thing is recorded on DVD.

Of course these affairs are a great excuse for a good lunch. Delicacies such as falafel, moutabel and kebabs are served followed by Arabic sweets such as baklava and *umm ali*, a delicately spiced bread and cream pudding. No wonder there is such a good turnout for us.

I host a goodbye tea party for my Arab women friends and colleagues, in a private room at the Ritz Carlton. Delicious tiered plates of sandwiches, scones and dainty cakes are served along with a selection of fine teas. We are on the top floor with a splendid view of the city and harbour. Once the waiters have departed the expensive abayas and veils are thrown off and I can see my friends' colourful attire and glossy long hair for the first time. I ask them about the segregation of the sexes at weddings and parties,

"It is better," Mona replies. "They have their chat and we have ours. We prefer to be separate."

I could never pretend that these are close friendships but everyone promises to keep in touch via email. Our abiding memories of our time in Qatar are of the warmth, humour and generosity of our Arab colleagues. Not that they are straightforward. Lionel once said to Noora, his secretary:

"You know what? I think I am gradually gaining their trust."

"No chance," she barked, "They don't even trust each other!"

Suddenly it is all over. I kiss Lionel good-bye then rush up to our hotel room to see his car racing over the causeway towards the airport at the other end of the city. I am alone in Doha. It is November and we had lived here for 800 days. Four weeks later, it is my turn to get into the limo and leave for the last time. Even then there is always a worry that they might not let me go. As I go through passport control, the officer scrutinises me, then my passport … then stops. My heart misses a beat.

"You have e-gate," he says. "You could have gone through the electronic system."

I just smile wanly whereupon he stamps my passport and I am through.

The great adventure is over. I am going home.

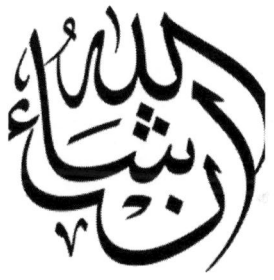

AUTHOR'S NOTE AND ACKNOWLEDGEMENTS

I would like to thank the many people who unwittingly helped shape the narrative of this book. Many of the names have been changed.

I am enormously grateful to my editor and publisher Amanda Field.

The readers of my original blog from Qatar were instrumental in encouraging my writing. I hope no one has been left out and there is an occasional addition of others who became involved once I had returned home. Many thanks to Angela and Jeremy Ames, Angelique Beling, Jane Bell, Clare Bennet, Anthea Bishop, Barbara Buckenham, Gemma Buckenham, Harry Bucknall, Antonia Calogeras, Kate Cameron, Suzanne Coates, Colin Coles, Michelle Coles, Jane and Ernest Crean, Diana and Steve Delia, Rebecca and Will Dobson, Debra Elliot, Ana Estruch, Emily and Peter Fabricius, Tim Fallon, Kathy Feest, John Gordon, Barbara Halliday, Ian and Shane Hamilton, Lynne Hansell, Amanda Havard, Edward Hill, Felicity Hill, Paula Hunt, Anna and Jonathan Jarvis, Marie Johnson, Sian and

Richard Jones, Alison Keightley, Charlotte Lampard, Nicola and Fred Latino, Michelle and Chris Lobo, Rosie Lusznat, Susie and Magnus McLaren, Sue and Bob Musselwhite, Jonathan Nash, Vicky Osgood, Finian O'Sullivan, Gora and Kate Pathak, Moira Phillips, Julia Pokora, Charley Ryan, Jane Reasbeck, Sally and Paul Sadler, Aileen Sced, Sarah Stevenson, Sharon and Denis Stubley, Lunar Summers, Ann and John Symes, John Tanzer, Stella and Peter Vaines, Frances and Michael Von Bertele, Sarah Vickers, Octavia Wayne, Abi and Steven Webber, Diana Wellesley, Rachel and Peter Wells, Lizzie and John Wilson, Jane Young and Tim Young.

The cover photograph of the author was taken by Maddie Attenborough of East Street Studio, Alresford, Hampshire; and the photograph opposite the *Introduction* is by Richard Jones.